An Introduction to Forensic Genetics

An Introduction to Forensic Genetics

Second Edition

William Goodwin

University of Central Lancashire, Preston, Lancashire, England, UK

Adrian Linacre

Flinders University, Adelaide, South Australia, Australia

Sibte Hadi

University of Central Lancashire, Preston, Lancashire, England, UK

A John Wiley & Sons, Ltd., Publication

This edition first published 2011, © 2011 by John Wiley & Sons Ltd

Wiley-Blackwell is an imprint of John Wiley & Sons, formed by the merger of Wiley's global Scientific, Technical and Medical business with Blackwell Publishing.

Registered office: John Wiley & Sons Ltd, The Atrium, Southern Gate, Chichester, West Sussex, PO19 8SQ, UK

Editorial Offices:
9600 Garsington Road, Oxford, OX4 2DQ, UK
The Atrium, Southern Gate, Chichester, West Sussex, PO19 8SQ, UK
111 River Street, Hoboken, NJ 07030-5774, USA

For details of our global editorial offices, for customer services and for information about how to apply for permission to reuse the copyright material in this book please see our website at www.wiley.com/wiley-blackwell

The right of the author to be identified as the author of this work has been asserted in accordance with the UK Copyright, Designs and Patents Act 1988.

Library of Congress Cataloguing-in-Publication Data

Goodwin, William, Dr.
  An introduction to forensic genetics / William Goodwin, Adrian Linacre, Sibte Hadi. – 2nd ed.
    p. ; cm.
  Includes bibliographical references and index.
  ISBN 978-0-470-71018-0 (cloth) – ISBN 978-0-470-71019-7 (pbk.)
  1. Forensic genetics. I. Linacre, Adrian. II. Hadi, Sibte. III. Title.
  [DNLM: 1. Forensic Genetics–methods. 2. DNA Fingerprinting. 3. Microsatellite Repeats. W 700]
  RA1057.5.G67 2011
  614′.1–dc22

                                                                        2010033354

A catalogue record for this book is available from the British Library.

This book is published in the following electronic format: ePDF: 978-0-470-97307-3

Set in 10.5/12.5 Times by Laserwords Private Limited, Chennai, India

First Impression   2011

Contents

Foreword

Essentials of forensic science

The world of forensic science is changing at a very fast pace. This is in terms of the provision of forensic science services, the development of technologies and knowledge and the interpretation of analytical and other data as it is applied within forensic practice. Practising forensic scientists are constantly striving to deliver the very best for the judicial process and as such need a reliable and robust knowledge base within their diverse disciplines. It is hoped that this book series will provide a resource by which such knowledge can be underpinned for both students and practitioners of forensic science alike.

The Forensic Science Society is the professional body for forensic practitioners in the United Kingdom. The Society was founded in 1959 and gained professional body status in 2006. The Society is committed to the development of the forensic sciences in all of its many facets, and in particular to the delivery of highly professional and worthwhile publications within these disciplines through ventures such as this book series.

Dr Niamh Nic Daéid
Reader in Forensic Science, University of Strathlcyde, Glasgow, Scotland, UK
UK Series Editor

Preface

It is strange to consider that the use of DNA in forensic science has been with us since 1985 and, although a relatively new discipline, it has impacted greatly on the criminal justice system and society as a whole. It is routinely the case that DNA figures in the media, in both real cases and fictional scenarios. The increased interest in forensic science has led to a burgeoning of university courses with modules in forensic science. This book is aimed at undergraduate students studying courses or modules in Forensic Genetics.

We have attempted to take the reader through the process of DNA profiling from the collection of biological evidence to the evaluation and presentation of genetic evidence. Although each chapter can stand alone, the order of chapters is designed to take the reader through the sequential steps in the generation of a DNA profile. The emphasis is on the use of short tandem repeat (STR) loci in human identification as this is currently the preferred technique. Following on from the process of generating a DNA profile, we have attempted to describe in accessible terms how a DNA profile is interpreted and evaluated. In addition, databases of DNA profiles have been developed in many countries and hence there is need to examine their use. While the focus of the book is on STR analysis, chapters on lineage markers and single nucleotide polymorphisms (SNPs) are also provided. A new Chapter has also been added to this edition that provides an overview of DNA profiling of non-human species.

As the field of forensic science and in particular DNA profiling moves onwards at a rapid pace, there are few introductory texts that cover the current state of this science. We are aware that there is a range of texts available that cover specific aspects of DNA profiling and where there this is the case, we direct readers to these books, papers or websites.

We hope that the readers of this book will gain an appreciation of both the underlying principles and the application of forensic genetics.

Preface to first edition

It is strange to consider that the use of DNA in forensic science has been with us for just over 20 years and, while a relatively new discipline, it has impacted greatly on the criminal justice system and society as a whole. It is routinely the case that DNA figures in the media, in both real cases and fictional scenarios.

The increased interest in forensic science has led to a burgeoning of university courses with modules in forensic science. This book is aimed at undergraduate students studying courses or modules in Forensic Genetics.

We have attempted to take the reader through the process of DNA profiling from the collection of biological evidence to the evaluation and presentation of genetic evidence. While each chapter can stand alone, the order of chapters is designed to take the reader throught the sequential steps in the generation of a DNA profile. The emphasis is on the use of short tandem repeat (STR) loci in human identification as this is currently the preferred technique. Following on from the process of generating a DNA profile, we have attempted to describe in accessible terms how a DNA profile is interpreted and evaluated. Databases of DNA profiles have been developed in many countries and hence there is need to examine their use. While the focus of the book is on STR analysis, chapters on lineage markers and single nucleotide polymorphisms (SNPs) are also provided.

As the field of forensic science and in particular DNA profiling moves onward at a rapid pace, there are few introductory texts that cover the current state of this science. We are aware that there is a range of texts available that cover specific aspects of DNA profiling and where there this is the case, we direct readers to these books, papers or web sites.

We hope that the readers of this book will gain an appreciation of both the underlying principles and application of forensic genetics.

1 Introduction to forensic genetics

The development and application of genetics has revolutionized forensic science. In 1984, the analysis of polymorphic regions of DNA produced what was termed 'a DNA fingerprint' [1]. The following year, at the request of the United Kingdom Home Office, DNA profiling was successfully applied to casework when it was used to resolve an immigration dispute [2]. In 1986, DNA evidence was used for the first time in a criminal case involving the murder of two young women in Leicestershire, UK: DNA analysis exonerated one individual who had confessed to one of the murders, and following a mass screen of approximately 5000 individuals, identified Colin Pitchfork as the murderer. He was convicted in January 1988 [3].[1]

Following on from early success in both civil and criminal cases, the use of genetics was rapidly adopted by the forensic community and now plays an important role worldwide in both the investigation of crime and in relationship testing. The scope and scale of DNA analysis in forensic science is set to continue expanding for the foreseeable future.

Forensic genetics

The work of the forensic geneticist will vary widely depending on the laboratory and country that they work in, and can involve the analysis of material recovered from a scene of crime, kinship testing and the identification of human remains. In some cases, it can even be used for the analysis of DNA from plants [6–18]; animals [19–36] including insects [37–60]; and microorganisms [61–67]. The focus of this book is the analysis of biological material that is recovered from the scene of crime – this is central to the work of most forensic laboratories. Kinship testing will be dealt with separately in Chapter 11 and a brief introduction is given to the testing of non-human material in Chapter 14.

Forensic laboratories receive material that has been recovered from scenes of crime, and reference samples from both suspects and victims. The role of forensic genetics within the investigative process is to compare samples recovered from crime

[1] Note: The first convictions in criminal cases came in 1987, when DNA evidence played an important role in the conviction of two rapists: Robert Melias in the UK and Tommy Lee Andrews in the USA [4, 5].

An Introduction to Forensic Genetics Second Edition   William Goodwin, Adrian Linacre and Sibte Hadi
© 2011 John Wiley & Sons, Ltd

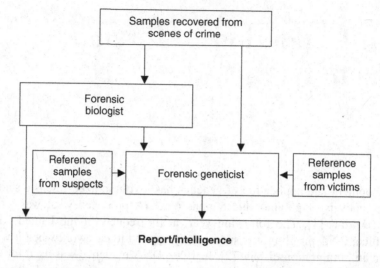

Figure 1.1   The role of the forensic geneticist is to assess whether samples recovered from a crime scene match to a suspect. Reference samples are provided from suspects and also victims of crime

scenes with suspects and possibly victims, resulting in a report that can be presented in court or intelligence that may inform an investigation (Figure 1.1).

Several stages are involved in the analysis of genetic evidence (Figure 1.2) and each of these is covered in detail in the following chapters. In some organizations one person will be responsible for collecting the evidence, the biological and genetic analysis of samples and ultimately presenting the results to a court of law. However, the trend in many larger organizations is for individuals to be responsible for only a very specific task within the process, such as the extraction of DNA from the evidential material or the analysis and interpretation of DNA profiles that have been generated by other scientists, or just reporting the findings.

A brief history of forensic genetics

In 1900 Karl Landsteiner described the ABO blood grouping system and observed that individuals could be placed into different groups based on their blood type. This was the first step in the development of forensic haemogenetics. Following on from this, numerous blood group markers and soluble blood serum protein markers were characterized and could be analysed in combination to produce highly discriminatory profiles. The serological techniques were a powerful tool but were limited in many forensic cases by the amount of biological material that was required to provide highly discriminating results. Proteins are also prone to degradation on exposure to the environment.

In the 1960s and 1970s, developments in molecular biology, including restriction enzymes, Sanger sequencing [68] and Southern blotting [69], enabled scientists to examine DNA sequences. By 1978, DNA polymorphisms could be detected using

Figure 1.2 Processes involved in generating a DNA profile following a crime. Some types of material, in particular blood and semen, are often characterized before DNA is extracted, allowing the DNA evidence to be linked to a cell type and possible transfer mechanism

Southern blotting [70] and in 1980 the analysis of the first highly polymorphic locus was reported, where the polymorphism was caused by differences in the lengths of the alleles [71].

It was not until September 1984 that Alec Jeffreys realized the potential forensic application of the minisatellite loci [1, 72, 73]. The technique developed by Jeffreys entailed extracting DNA and cutting it with a restriction enzyme before carrying out agarose gel electrophoresis, Southern blotting and probe hybridization to detect the polymorphic loci. The end result was a series of black bands on X-ray film, which was called a DNA fingerprint (Figure 1.3).

(a)   (b)

Figure 1.3   (a) The first ever DNA fingerprint, produced in Alec Jeffreys' laboratory on the 10th September 1984. It shows the banding pattern from a mother, child, and father: the bands in the child's profile can be attributed to either the mother or the father. (b) Profiles from a mother, a tested child (TC) (Immigration Officials in the UK did not believe that the boy was the biological son of the mother) and three of the mother's undisputed children (UD 1-3): the results demonstrated that the tested child was indeed the biological son of the woman and was therefore allowed to stay in the UK [2]. (Images provided by Sir Prof Alec Jeffreys, Department of Genetics, University of Leicester, UK)

With the first DNA fingerprints the multi-locus probes (MLPs) detected several minisatellite loci simultaneously, leading to the multiple band patterns. While the multi-banded fingerprints were highly informative they were difficult to interpret. New probes were designed that were specific to one locus (single locus probes, SLPs) and therefore produced only one or two bands for each individual [74] (Figure 1.4).

Minisatellite analysis was a powerful tool but suffered from several limitations: a relatively large amount of DNA was required; it would not work with degraded DNA; comparison between laboratories was difficult; and the analysis was time consuming. Even so, the use of minisatellite analysis, using SLPs, was common for several years [75] until it was replaced by polymerase chain reaction (PCR)-based systems.

A critical development in the history of forensic genetics came with the advent of a process that can amplify specific regions of DNA – the PCR (see Chapter 5). The PCR process was conceptualized in 1983 by Kary Mullis, a chemist working for the Cetus Corporation in the USA [76]. The development of PCR has had a profound effect on all aspects of molecular biology including forensic genetics, and in recognition of the significance of the development of the technique Kary Mullis was awarded the Nobel Prize for Chemistry in 1993.

Figure 1.4 Minisatellite analysis using a single locus probe: ladders were run alongside the tested samples that allowed the size of the DNA fragments to be estimated. A control sample labelled K562 was analysed along with the tested samples

The PCR increases the sensitivity of DNA analysis to the point where DNA profiles can be generated from just a few cells, reduces the time required to produce a profile, can be used with degraded DNA and allows just about any polymorphism in the genome to be analysed.

The first application of PCR in a forensic case involved the analysis of single nucleotide polymorphisms in the human leukocyte antigen (HLA)-DQα locus (part of the major histocompatibility complex (MHC)) [77] (see Chapter 12). This was soon followed by the analysis of short tandem repeats (STRs), which are currently the most commonly used genetic markers in forensic science (see Chapters 6–8). The rapid development of technology for analysing DNA includes advances in DNA extraction and quantification methodology, the development of commercial PCR-based typing kits and equipment for detecting DNA polymorphisms.

In addition to technical advances, another important part of the development of DNA profiling that has had an impact on the whole field of forensic science is quality assurance. The admissibility of DNA evidence was seriously challenged in the USA in 1989 – *People* v. *Castro* [78]; this and subsequent cases in many countries have resulted in increased levels of standardization and quality assurance in forensic genetics and other areas of forensic science. As a result, the accreditation of both laboratories and individuals is an increasingly important issue in forensic science. The combination of technical advances, high levels of standardization and quality assurance have led to forensic DNA analysis being recognized as a robust and reliable forensic tool.

References

1. Jeffreys, A.J. Wilson, V. and Thein, S.L. (1985) Individual-specific fingerprints of human DNA. *Nature*, **316**, 76–79.
2. Jeffreys, A.J., Brookfield, J.F.Y. and Semenoff, R. (1985) Positive identification of an immigration test-case using human DNA fingerprints. *Nature*, **317**, 818–819.
3. Seton, C. (1988) Life for Sex Killer who Sent Decoy to Take Genetic Test. *The Times* (London).
4. McCarthy, M. (1987) Rapist in Genetic Fingerprint Case Jailed for 8 Years. *The Times* (London).
5. Andrews, T.L. (1987) State v. Andrews. 9th Cir. Ct, Orange Co., Fla, Div 15.
6. Kress, W.J., Wurdack, K.J., Zimmer, E.A., Weigt, L.A. and Janzen, D.H. (2005) Use of DNA barcodes to identify flowering plants. *Proceedings of the National Academy of Sciences of the United States of America*, **102**, 8369–8374.
7. Linacre, A. and Thorpe, J. (1998) Detection and identification of cannabis by DNA. *Forensic Science International*, **91**, 71–76.
8. Bless, C., Palmeter, H. and Wallace, M.M. (2006) Identification of Acer rubrum using amplified fragment length polymorphism. *Journal of Forensic Sciences*, **51**, 31–38.
9. Cowan, R.S., Chase, M.W., Kress, W.J. and Savolainen, V. (2006) 300,000 species to identify: problems, progress, and prospects in DNA barcoding of land plants. *Taxon*, **55**, 611–616.
10. Craft, K.J., Owens, J.D. and Ashley, M.V. (2007) Application of plant DNA markers in forensic botany: genetic comparison of Quercus evidence leaves to crime scene trees using microsatellites. *Forensic Science International*, **165**, 64–70.
11. Datwyler, S.L. and Weiblen, G.D. (2006) Genetic variation in hemp and marijuana (*Cannabis sativa* L.) according to amplified fragment length polymorphisms. *Journal of Forensic Sciences*, **51**, 371–375.
12. Ferri, G., Alu, M., Corradini, B. and Beduschi, G. (2009) Forensic botany: species identification of botanical trace evidence using a multigene barcoding approach. *International Journal of Legal Medicine*, **123**, 395–401.
13. Finkeldey, R., Leinemann, L. and Gailing, O. (2010) Molecular genetic tools to infer the origin of forest plants and wood. *Applied Microbiology and Biotechnology*, **85**, 1251–1258.
14. Howard, C., Gilmore, S., Robertson, J. and Peakall, R. (2008) Developmental validation of a *Cannabis sativa* STIR multiplex system for forensic analysis. *Journal of Forensic Sciences*, **53**, 1061–1067.
15. Howard, C., Gilmore, S., Robertson, J. and Peakall, R. (2009) A *Cannabis sativa* STR genotype database for Australian seizures: forensic applications and limitations. *Journal of Forensic Sciences*, **54**, 556–563.
16. Kojoma, M., Seki, H., Yoshida, S. and Muranaka, T. (2006) DNA polymorphisms in the tetrahydrocannabinolic acid (THCA) synthase gene in "drug-type" and "fiber-type" *Cannabis sativa* L. *Forensic Science International*, **159**, 132–140.
17. Kress, W.J., Erickson, D.L., Jones, F.A., Swenson, N.G., Perez, R., Sanjur, O. *et al.* (2009) Plant DNA barcodes and a community phylogeny of a tropical forest dynamics plot in Panama. *Proceedings of the National Academy of Sciences of the United States of America*, **106**, 18621–18626.
18. Tsai, L.C., Yu, Y.C., Hsieh, H.M., Wang, J.C., Linacre, A. and Lee, J.C.I. (2006) Species identification using sequences of the trnL intron and the trnL-trnF IGS of chloroplast genome among popular plants in Taiwan. *Forensic Science International*, **164**, 193–200.
19. Hebert, P.D.N., Ratnasingham, S., deWaard, J.R. (2003) Barcoding animal life: cytochrome c oxidase subunit 1 divergences among closely related species. *Proceedings of the Royal Society of London Series B: Biological Sciences*, **270**, S96–S99.

20. Parson, W., Pegoraro, K., Niederstatter, H., Foger, M. and Steinlechner, M. (2000) Species identification by means of the cytochrome b gene. *International Journal of Legal Medicine*, **114**, 23–28.

21. Eichmann, C. and Parson, W. (2007) Molecular characterization of the canine mitochondrial DNA control region for forensic applications. *International Journal of Legal Medicine*, **121**, 411–416.

22. Fernandes, C.A., Ginja, C., Pereira, I., Tenreiro, R., Bruford, M.W. and Santos-Reis, M. (2008) Species-specific mitochondrial DNA markers for identification of non-invasive samples from sympatric carnivores in the Iberian Peninsula. *Conservation Genetics*, **9**, 681–690.

23. Halverson, J.L. and Basten, C. (2005) Forensic DNA identification of animal-derived trace evidence: tools for linking victims and suspects. *Croatian Medical Journal*, **46**, 598–605.

24. Hellmann, A.P., Rohleder, U., Eichmann, C., Pfeiffer, I., Parson, W. and Schleenbecker, U. (2006) A proposal for standardization in forensic canine DNA typing: allele nomenclature of six canine-specific STR loci. *Journal of Forensic Sciences*, **51**, 274–281.

25. Hsieh, H.M., Huang, L.H., Tsaim L.C., Liu, C.L., Kuo, Y.C., Hsiao, C.T. *et al.* (2006) Species identification of Kachuga tecta using the cytochrome b gene. *Journal of Forensic Sciences*, **51**, 52–56.

26. Imaizumi, K., Akutsu, T., Miyasaka, S. and Yoshino, M. (2007) Development of species identification tests targeting the 16S ribosomal RNA coding region in mitochondrial DNA. *International Journal of Legal Medicine*, **121**, 184–191.

27. Lee, J.C.I., Tsai, L.C., Yang, C.Y., Liu, C.L., Huang, L.H., Linacre, A. *et al.* (2006) DNA profiling of shahtoosh. *Electrophoresis*, **27**, 3359–3362.

28. Magnussen, J.E., Pikitch, E.K., Clarke, S.C., Nicholson, C., Hoelzel, A.R., Shivji, M.S. (2007) Genetic tracking of basking shark products in international trade. *Animal Conservation*, **10**, 199–207.

29. Meganathan, P.R., Dubey, B., Haque, I. (2009) Molecular identification of crocodile species using novel primers for forensic analysis. *Conservation Genetics*, **10**, 767–770.

30. Melton, T. and Holland, C. (2007) Routine forensic use of the mitochondrial 12S ribosomal RNA gene for species identification. *Journal of Forensic Sciences*, **52**, 1305–1307.

31. Menotti-Raymond, M.A., Dubey, B. and Haque, I. (2005) An STIR forensic typing system for genetic individualization of domestic cat (Felis catus) samples. *Journal of Forensic Sciences*, **50**, 1061–1070.

32. Nakaki, S., Hino, D., Miyoshi, M., Nakayama, H., Moriyoshi, H., Morikawa, T. *et al.* (2007) Study of animal species (human, dog and cat) identification using a multiplex single-base primer extension reaction in the cytochrome b gene. *Forensic Science International*, **173**, 97–102.

33. van Asch, B., Alves, C., Gusmao, L., Pereira, V., Pereira, F. and Amorim, A. (2009) A new autosomal STR nineplex for canine identification and parentage testing. *Electrophoresis*, **30**, 417–423.

34. van Asch, B., Pinheiro, R., Pereira, R., Alves, C., Pereira, V., Pereira, F. *et al.* (2010) A framework for the development of STR genotyping in domestic animal species: Characterization and population study of 12 canine X-chromosome loci. *Electrophoresis*, **31**, 303–308.

35. Wan, Q.H. and Fang, S.G. (2003) Application of species-specific polymerase chain reaction in the forensic identification of tiger species. *Forensic Science International*, **131**, 75–78.

36. Webb, K.M. and Allard, M.W. (2009) Mitochondrial genome DNA analysis of the domestic dog: identifying informative SNPs outside of the control region. *Journal of Forensic Sciences*, **54**, 275–288.

37. Mazzanti, M., Alessandrini, F., Tagliabracci, A., Wells, J.D. and Campobasso, C.P. (2010) DNA degradation and genetic analysis of empty puparia: genetic identification limits in forensic entomology. *Forensic Science International*, **195**, 99–102.

38. Chen, W.Y., Hung, T.H. and Shiao, S.F. (2004) Molecular identification of forensically important blow fly species (Diptera: Calliphoridae) in Taiwan. *Journal of Medical Entomology*, **41**, 47–57.

39. Desmyter, S. and Gosselin, M. (2009) COI sequence variability between Chrysomyinae of forensic interest. *Forensic Science International-Genetics*, **3**, 89–95.

40. DiZinno, J.A., Lord, W.D., Collins-Morton, M.B., Wilson, M.R. and Goff, M.L. (2002) Mitochondrial DNA sequencing of beetle larvae (Nitidulidae: Omosita) recovered from human bone. *Journal of Forensic Sciences*, **47**, 1337–1339.

41. Draber-Monko, A., Malewski, T., Pomorski, J., Los, M. and Slipinski, P. (2009) On the morphology and mitochondrial DNA barcoding of the flesh fly sarcophaga (Liopygia) argyrostoma (Robineau-Desvoidy, 1830) (Diptera: Sarcophagidae) – an important species in forensic entomology. *Annales Zoologici*, **59**, 465–493.

42. Gariepy, T.D., Kuhlmann, U., Gillott, C. and Erlandson, M. (2007) Parasitoids, predators and PCR: the use of diagnostic molecular markers in biological control of Arthropods. *Journal of Applied Entomology*, **131**, 225–240.

43. Harvey, M.L., Dadour, I.R. and Gaudieri, S. (2003) Mitochondrial DNA cytochrome oxidase I gene: potential for distinction between immature stages of some forensically important fly species (Diptera) in western Australia. *Forensic Science International*, **131**, 134–139.

44. Harvey, M.L., Gaudieri, S., Villet, M.H. and Dadour, I.R. (2008) A global study of forensically significant calliphorids: implications for identification. *Forensic Science International*, **177**, 66–76.

45. Harvey, M.L., Mansell, M.W., Villet, M.H. and Dadour, I.R. (2003) Molecular identification of some forensically important blowflies of southern Africa and Australia. *Medical and Veterinary Entomology*, **17**, 363–369.

46. Malgorn, Y. and Coquoz, R. (1999) DNA typing for identification of some species of Calliphoridae – an interest in forensic entomology. *Forensic Science International*, **102**, 111–119.

47. Nelson, L.A., Wallman, J.F. and Dowton, M. (2007) Using COI barcodes to identify forensically and medically important blowflies. *Medical and Veterinary Entomology*, **21**, 44–52.

48. Nelson, L.A., Wallman, J.F. and Dowton, M. (2008) Identification of forensically important Chrysomya (Diptera: Calliphoridae) species using the second ribosomal internal transcribed spacer (ITS2). *Forensic Science International*, **177**, 238–247.

49. Park, S.H., Zhang, Y., Piao, H., Yu, D.H., Jeong, H.J. and Yoo, G.Y. (2009) Use of Cytochrome c Oxidase Subunit I (COI) nucleotide sequences for identification of the Korean Luciliinae fly species (Diptera: Calliphoridae) in forensic investigations. *Journal of Korean Medical Science*, **24**, 1058–1063.

50. Park, S.H., Zhang, Y., Piao, H., Yu, D.H., Jeong, H.J., Yoo, G.Y. *et al.* (2009) Sequences of the Cytochrome C Oxidase Subunit I (COI) gene are suitable for species identification of Korean Calliphorinae flies of forensic importance (Diptera: Calliphoridae). *Journal of Forensic Sciences*, **54**, 1131–1134.

51. Reibe, S., Schmitz, J. and Madea, B. (2009) Molecular identification of forensically important blowfly species (Diptera: Calliphoridae) from Germany. *Parasitology Research*, **106**, 257–261.

52. Rodrigues, R.A., de Azeredo-Espin, A.M.L. and Torres, T.T. (2009) Microsatellite markers for population genetic studies of the blowfly Chrysomya putoria (Diptera: Calliphoridae). *Memorias Do Instituto Oswaldo Cruz*, **104**, 1047–1050.

53. Schroeder, H., Klotzbach, H., Elias, S., Augustin, C. and Pueschel, K. (2003) Use of PCR-RFLP for differentiation of calliphorid larvae (Diptera, Calliphoridae) on human corpses. *Forensic Science International*, **132**, 76–81.

54. Thyssen, P.J., Lessinger, A.C., Azeredo-Espin, A.M.L. and Linhares, A.X. (2005) The value of PCR-RFLP molecular markers for the differentiation of immature stages of two necrophagous flies (Diptera: Calliphoridae) of potential forensic importance. *Neotropical Entomology*, **34**, 777–783.

55. Wallman, J.F. and Adams, M. (2001) The forensic application of allozyme electrophoresis to the identification of blowfly larvae (Diptera: Calliphoridae) in southern Australia. *Journal of Forensic Sciences*, **46**, 681–684.

56. Wallman, J.F. and Donnellan, S.C. (2001) The utility of mitochondrial DNA sequences for the identification of forensically important blowflies (Diptera: Calliphoridae) in southeastern Australia. *Forensic Science International*, **120**, 60–67.

57. Wells, J.D., Pape, T. and Sperling, F.A.H. (2001) DNA-based identification and molecular systematics of forensically important sarcophagidae (diptera). *Journal of Forensic Sciences*, **46**, 1098–1102.

58. Wells, J.D. and Sperling, F.A.H. (2001) DNA-based identification of forensically important Chrysomyinae (Diptera: Calliphoridae). *Forensic Science International*, **120**, 110–115.

59. Wells, J.D. and Stevens, J.R. (2008) Application of DNA-based methods in forensic entomology. *Annual Review of Entomology*, **53**, 103–120.

60. Zehner, R., Amendt, J., Schutt, S., Sauer, J., Krettek, R. and Povolny, D. (2004) Genetic identification of forensically important flesh flies (Diptera: Sarcophagidae). *International Journal of Legal Medicine*, **118**, 245–247.

61. Hoffmaster, A.R., Fitzgerald, C.C., Ribot, E., Mayer, L.W. and Popovic, T. (2002) Molecular subtyping of Bacillus anthracis and the 2001 bioterrorism-associated anthrax outbreak, United States. *Emerging Infectious Diseases*, **8**, 1111–1116.

62. Bhattacharjee, Y. and Enserink, M. (2008) Anthrax investigation – FBI discusses microbial forensics – but key questions remain unanswered. *Science*, **321**, 1026–1027.

63. Budowle, B., Schutzer, S.E., Einseln, A., Kelley, L.C., Walsh, A.C., Smith, J.A.L., *et al.* (2003) Building microbial forensics as a response to bioterrorism. *Science*, **301**, 1852–1853.

64. Cummings, C.A. and Relman, D.A. (2002) Genomics and microbiology – microbial forensics – "Cross-examining pathogens". *Science*, **296**, 1976–1979.

65. Enserink, M. (2008) Anthrax investigation – full-genome sequencing paved the way from spores to a suspect. *Science*, **321**, 898–899.

66. Keim, P., Pearson, T. and Okinaka, R. (2008) Microbial forensics: DNA fingerprinting of Bacillus anthracis (Anthrax). *Analytical Chemistry*, **80**, 4791–4799.

67. Pattnaik, P. and Jana, A.M. (2005) Microbial forensics: applications in bioterrorism. *Environmental Forensics*, **6**, 197–204.

68. Sanger, F., Nicklen, S. and Coulson, A.R. (1977) DNA sequencing with chain-terminating inhibitors. *Proceedings of the National Academy of Sciences of the United States of America*, **74**, 5463–5467.

69. Southern, E.M. (1975) Detection of specific sequences among DNA fragments separated by gel electrophoresis. *Journal of Molecular Biology*, **98**, 503–517.

70. Kan, Y.W. and Dozy, A.M. (1978) Polymorphism of DNA sequence adjacent to human B-globin structural gene: relationship to sickle mutation. *Proceedings of the National Academy of Science of the United States of America*, **75**, 5631–5635.

71. Wyman, A.R. and White, R. (1980) A highly polymorphic locus in human DNA. *Proceedings of the National Academy of Science of the United States of America*, **77**, 6754–6758.

72. Jeffreys, A.J. and Wilson, V. (1985) Hypervariable regions in human DNA. *Genetical Research*, **45**, 213–213.

73. Gill, P., Jeffreys, A.J. and Werrett, D.J. (1985) Forensic application of DNA 'fingerprints'. *Nature*, **318**, 577–579.

74. Wong, Z., Wilson, V., Patel, I., Povey, S., Jeffreys, A.J. (1987) Characterization of a panel of highly variable minisatellites cloned from human DNA. *Annals of Human Genetics*, **51**, 269–288.

75. Hallenberg, C. and Morling, N. (2002) A report of the 2000 and 2001 paternity testing workshops of the English speaking working group of the international society for forensic genetics. *Forensic Science International*, **129**, 43–50.

76. Saiki, R.K., Scharf, S., Faloona, F., Mullis, K.B., Horn, G.T., Erlich, H.A. *et al.* (1985) Enzymatic amplification of beta-globin genomic sequences and restriction site analysis for diagnosis of sickle-cell anemia. *Science*, **230**, 1350–1354.

77. Stoneking, M., Hedgecock, D., Higuchi, R.G., Vigilant, L. and Erlich, H.A. (1991) Population variation of human mtDNA control region sequences detected by enzymatic amplification and sequence-specific oligonucleotide probes. *American Journal of Human Genetics*, **48**, 370–382.

78. Patton, S.M. (1990) DNA fingerprinting: the Castro case. *Harvard Journal of Law and Technology*, **3**, 223–240.

2 DNA structure and the genome

Each person's genome contains a large amount of DNA that is a potential target for DNA profiling. The selection of the particular region of polymorphic DNA to analyse can change with the individual case and also the technology that is available. In this chapter a brief description of the primary structure of the DNA molecule is provided along with an overview of the different categories of DNA that make up the human genome. The criteria that the forensic geneticist uses to select which loci to analyse are also discussed.

DNA structure

DNA has often been described as the 'blueprint of life', containing all the information that an organism requires in order to function and reproduce. The DNA molecule that carries out such a fundamental biological role is relatively simple. The basic building block of the DNA molecule is the nucleotide triphosphate (Figure 2.1a). This comprises a triphosphate group, a deoxyribose sugar (Figure 2.1b) and one of four bases (Figure 2.1c).

The information within the DNA 'blueprint' is coded by the sequence of the four different nitrogenous bases, adenine, guanine, thymine and cytosine, on the sugar–phosphate backbone (Figure 2.2a).

DNA normally exists as a double-stranded molecule that adopts a helical arrangement – first described by Watson and Crick in 1953 [1]. Each base is attracted to its complementary base: adenine always pairs with thymine and cytosine always pairs with guanine (Figure 2.2b).

Organization of DNA into chromosomes

Within each nucleated human cell there are two complete copies of the genome. The genome is 'the haploid genetic complement of a living organism' and in humans contains approximately 3 200 000 000 bp of information, which is organized into 23 chromosomes. Humans contain two sets of chromosomes – one version of each chromosome inherited from each parent giving a total of 46 chromosomes [2] (Figure 2.3).

An Introduction to Forensic Genetics Second Edition   William Goodwin, Adrian Linacre and Sibte Hadi
© 2011 John Wiley & Sons, Ltd

Figure 2.1 The DNA molecule is built up of deoxynucleotide 5′ triphosphates (a). The sugar (b) contains five carbon atoms (labelled C1–C5); one of four different types of nitrogenous base (c) is attached to the 1′ carbon, a hydroxyl group to the 3′ carbon and the phosphate group to the 5′ carbon. Adenine and guanine both have a double ring and are purines, whereas cytosine and thymine have a single ring and are pyrimidines

Figure 2.2 Nucleotides are joined together by phosphodiester bonds to form a single-stranded molecule (a). The DNA molecule in the cell is double-stranded (b) with two complementary single-stranded molecules held together by hydrogen bonds. Adenine and thymine form two hydrogen bonds while guanine and cytosine form three bonds

Figure 2.3 The male human karyotype pictured contains 46 chromosomes, 22 autosomes and the X and Y sex chromosomes – the female karyotype has two X chromosomes. The chromosomes have been labelled with fluorescent probes allowing them to be identified. (Image provided by Duncan Holdsworth, Westlakes Research Institute, University of Central Lancashire, UK)

Each chromosome contains one continuous strand of DNA, the largest – chromosome 1 – is approximately 250 000 000 bp long whereas the smallest – chromosome 22 – is approximately 50 000 000 bp [3–5]. In physical terms the chromosomes range in length from 73 mm to 14 mm. The chromosomes shown in Figure 2.3 are in the metaphase stage of the cell cycle and are highly condensed – when the cell is not undergoing division the chromosomes are less highly ordered and are more diffuse within the nucleus. To achieve the highly ordered chromosome structure, the DNA molecule is associated with histone proteins, which help the packaging and organization of the DNA into the ordered chromosome structure.

The structure of the human genome

Great advances have been made in our understanding of the human genome in recent years, in particular through the work of the Human Genome Project, which was officially started in 1990 with the central aim of decoding the entire genome. It involved a collaborative effort involving 20 centres in China, France, Germany, Great Britain, Japan and the United States. Draft sequences were produced in 2001,

Figure 2.4   The human genome can be classified into different types of DNA based on its structure and function. (Based on Jasinska and Krzyzosiak [11])

one by the Public Consortium and one by the private organization Celera Genomics, that covered 90% of the euchromatic DNA [4, 5]. This was followed by later versions that described the sequence of 99% of the euchromatic DNA with an accuracy of 99.99% [3]. The first genomes were composites made up from sequence data from different individuals; genomes of several individuals have now been decoded [6–10].

The genome can be divided into different categories of DNA based on the structure and function of the sequence (Figure 2.4).

Coding and regulatory sequence

The regions of DNA that encode and regulate the synthesis of proteins are called genes; at the latest estimate the human genome contains only 20 000–25 000 genes and only around 1.5% of the genome is directly involved in encoding for proteins [3–5]. Gene structure, sequence and activity are a focus of medical genetics because of the interest in genetic defects and the expression of genes within cells. Approximately 23.5% of the genome is classified as genic sequence, but does not encode proteins. The non-coding genic sequence contains several elements that are involved with the regulation of genes, including promoters, enhancers, repressors and polyadenylation signals; the majority of gene-related DNA, around 23%, is made up of introns, pseudogenes and gene fragments.

Extragenic DNA

Most of the genome, approximately 75%, is extragenic. Around 20% of the genome is single copy DNA, which in most cases does not have any known function, although some regions appear to be under evolutionary pressure and presumably play an important, but as yet unknown, role [12].

The largest portion of the genome – over 50% – is composed of repetitive DNA; 45% of the repetitive DNA is interspersed, with the repeat elements dispersed throughout the genome. The four most common types of interspersed repetitive element – short interspersed elements (SINEs), long interspersed elements (LINEs), long terminal repeats (LTRs) and DNA transposons – account for 45% of the genome [4, 13]. These repeat sequences are all derived through transposition. The most common interspersed repeat element is the *Alu* SINE; with over 1 million copies, the repeat is approximately 300 bp long and makes up around 10% of the genome. There is a similar number of LINE elements within the genome; the most common is LINE1, which is between 6 kb and 8 kb long, and is represented in the genome around 900 000 times; LINEs make up around 21% of the genome [4, 13]. The other class of repetitive element is tandemly repeated DNA. This can be separated into three different types: satellite DNA, minisatellites and microsatellites.

Genetic diversity of modern humans

The aim of using genetic analysis for forensic casework is to produce a DNA profile that is highly discriminating; the ideal would be to generate a DNA profile that is unique to each individual. This allows biological evidence from the scene of a crime to be matched to an individual with a high degree of confidence and can be very powerful forensic evidence.

The ability to produce highly discriminating profiles is dependent on individuals being different at the genetic level and, with the exception of identical twins, no two individuals have been found to have the same DNA. However, individuals, even ones who appear very different, are actually very similar at the genetic level. Indeed, if we compare the human genome to that of our closest animal cousin, the chimpanzee, with whom we shared a common ancestor around 6 million years ago, we find that our genomes have diverged by only around 5%; the DNA sequence has diverged by only 1.2% [14] and insertions and deletions in both human and chimpanzee genomes account for another 3.5% divergence [14, 15]. This means that we share 95% of our DNA with chimps! Modern humans have a much more recent common history, which has been dated using genetic and fossil data to around 150 000 years ago [16, 17]. In this limited time, nucleotide substitutions have led to an average of one difference every 1000 bases between every human chromosome, averaging one difference every 1250 bp [5, 18] – which means that we share around 99.9% of our genetic code with each other. Some additional variation is caused by insertions, deletions, length polymorphisms and segmental duplications of the genome [6–10, 19].

There have been attempts to define populations genetically based on their racial identity or geographical location, and while it has been possible to classify individuals genetically into broad racial/geographic groupings, it has been shown that most genetic variation, around 85%, can be attributed to differences between individuals within a population [20, 21]. Differences between regions tend to be geographic gradients (clines), with gradual changes in allele frequencies [22–27].

From a forensic point of view there is very little rationale in analysing the 99.9% of human DNA that is common between individuals. Fortunately, there are well-characterized regions within the genome that are variable between individuals and these have become the focus of forensic genetics.

The genome and forensic genetics

With advances in molecular biology techniques it is now possible to analyse any region within the 3.2 billion bases that make up the human genome. DNA loci that are to be used for forensic genetics should have some key properties; they should ideally:

- be highly polymorphic (varying widely between individuals);
- be easy and cheap to characterize;
- give profiles that are simple to interpret and easy to compare between laboratories;
- not be under any selective pressure; and
- have a low mutation rate.

Tandem repeats

Two important categories of tandem repeat have been used widely in forensic genetics: minisatellites, also referred to as variable number tandem repeats (VNTRs); and microsatellites, also referred to as STRs. The general structure of mini- and microsatellites is the same (Figures 2.5 and 2.6). Variation between different alleles is caused by a different number of the repeat unit, which in turn results in alleles that are of different lengths; it is for this reason that tandem repeat polymorphisms are also known as length polymorphisms.

| A-type CCCTATCCA | B-type CCCTCTCCA | Other repeat variant |
| C-type CCCTGTCCA | K-type CCCTAACCA | |

Figure 2.5 The structure of two minisatellite alleles found at the D1S7 locus [28]. The alleles are both relatively short containing 104 and 134 repeats; alleles at this locus can contain over 2000 repeats. The alleles are composed of several different variants of the 9 bp core repeat; this is a common feature of minisatellite alleles

Figure 2.6 The structure of a short tandem repeat. This example shows the structure of two alleles from the locus D8S1179.[1] The DNA either side of the core repeats is called flanking DNA. The alleles are named according to the number of repeats that they contain – hence alleles 8 and 10

Minisatellites

Minisatellites are located predominantly in the subtelomeric regions of chromosomes and have a core repeat sequence that ranges in size from 6 bp to 100 bp [30, 31]. The core repeats are represented in some alleles thousands of times; the variation in repeat number creates alleles that range in size from 500 bp to over 30 kb (Figure 2.5). The number of potential alleles can be very large: the D1S7 locus, for example has a relatively short and simple core repeat unit of 9 bp with alleles that range from approximately 1 kb to over 20 kb – which means that there are potentially over 2000 different alleles at this locus [28].

Minisatellites were the first polymorphisms used in DNA profiling [32, 33] and they were successfully used in forensic casework for several years. The use of minisatellites was, however, limited by the type of sample that could be successfully analysed, because a large amount of high molecular weight DNA was required. Interpreting minisatellite profiles could also be problematic. Their use in forensic genetics has now been replaced by microsatellites, which are also known as STRs.

Short tandem repeats

STRs are currently the most commonly analysed genetic polymorphism in forensic genetics. They were introduced into casework in the mid-1990s and are now the main tool for just about every forensic laboratory in the world – the vast majority of forensic genetic casework involves the analysis of STR polymorphisms.

There are thousands of STRs that can potentially be used for forensic analysis. STR loci are spread throughout the genome, including the 22 autosomal chromosomes and the X and Y sex chromosomes. They have a core unit of between 1 bp[2] and 6 bp and the alleles typically range from 50 bp to 300 bp. The majority of the loci that are used in forensic genetics are tetranucleotide repeats, which have a 4 bp repeat motif (Figure 2.6).

---

[1] Note: The considerations for describing STR structure have been documented by the International Society for Forensic Genetics (ISFG) [29].

[2] Note: STRs with repeating core units of one base pair are not used in forensic analysis.

5′-GATGGCA-3′	allele G
*	
5′-GATAGCA-3′	allele A

Figure 2.7 A single nucleotide polymorphism (SNP). Two alleles are shown which differ at one position indicated by the star: the fourth position in allele G is a guanine while in allele A it is an adenine. In most cases, the mutation event at the specific locus that creates a SNP is a unique event and only two different alleles (biallelic) are normally found

STRs satisfy all the requirements for a forensic marker: they are robust, leading to successful analysis of a wide range of biological material; the results generated in different laboratories are easily compared; they are highly discriminatory, especially when analysing a large number of loci simultaneously (multiplexing); they are very sensitive, requiring only a few cells for a successful analysis; it is relatively cheap and easy to generate STR profiles; and there is a large number of STRs throughout the genome that do not appear to be under any selective pressure.

Single nucleotide polymorphisms

The simplest type of polymorphism is the single nucleotide polymorphism (SNP): single base differences in the sequence of the DNA. The structure of a typical SNP polymorphism is illustrated in Figure 2.7.

SNPs are formed when errors (mutations) occur as the cell undergoes DNA replication during meiosis. Some regions of the genome are richer in SNPs than others [34].

SNPs normally have just two alleles, for example one allele with a guanine and one with an adenine. This is a purine for a purine, other common changes are between cytosine and thymine, both of which are pyrimidines. SNPs therefore are not highly polymorphic and do not fit with the ideal properties of DNA polymorphisms for forensic analysis. However, SNPs are so abundant throughout the genome that it is theoretically possible to type hundreds of them. This can result in very high combined power of discrimination. It is estimated that to achieve the same discriminatory power that is achieved using 10 STRs, 50–80 SNPs would have to be analysed [35, 36]. With current technology, this is much more difficult than analysing 10 to 15 STR loci.

With the exception of the analysis of mitochondrial DNA (see Chapter 13), SNPs have not been used widely in forensic science to date, and the dominance of tandem repeated DNA will continue for the foreseeable future [37]. SNPs are however finding a number of niche applications in forensic science (see Chapter 12).

WWW resources

The Human Genome Project Information: a website funded by the U.S. Department of Energy which along with and the National Institutes of Health coordinated the project. Contains resources on all aspects of the Human Genome Project. http://www.ornl.gov/sci/techresources/HumanGenome/home.shtml

References

1. Watson, J. and Crick, F. (1953) A structure for deoxyribose nucleic acid. *Nature*, **171**, 737–738.
2. Tjio, J.H. and Levèn, A. (1956) The chromosome number of man. *Hereditas*, **42**, 1–6.
3. Collins, F.S., Lander, E.S., Rogers, J. and Waterston, R.H. (2004) Finishing the euchromatic sequence of the human genome. *Nature*, **431**, 931–945.
4. Lander, E.S., Linton, L.M., Birren, B., Nusbaum, C., Zody, M.C., Baldwin, J. *et al.* (2001) Initial sequencing and analysis of the human genome. *Nature*, **409**, 860–921.
5. Venter, J.C., Adams, M.D., Myers, E.W., Li, P.W., Mural, R.J. and Sutton, G.G. (2001) The sequence of the human genome. *Science*, **291**, 1304–1351.
6. Levy, S., Sutton, G., Ng, P.C., Feuk, L., Halpern, A.L. and Walenz, B.P. (2007) The diploid genome sequence of an individual human. *Plos Biology*, **5**, 2113–2144.
7. Schuster, S.C., Miller, W., Ratan, A., Tomsho, L.P., Giardine, B., Kasson, L.R. *et al.* (2010) Complete Khoisan and Bantu genomes from southern Africa. *Nature*, **463**, 943–947.
8. Wang, J., Wang, W., Li, R.Q., Li, Y.R., Tian, G., Goodman, L. *et al.* (2008) The diploid genome sequence of an Asian individual. *Nature*, **456**, 60–61.
9. Wheeler, D.A., Srinivasan, M., Egholm, M., Shen, Y., Chen, L., McGuire, A. *et al.* (2008) The complete genome of an individual by massively parallel DNA sequencing. *Nature*, **452**, 872–875.
10. Bentley, D.R., Balasubramanian, S., Swerdlow, H.P., Smith, G.P., Milton, J., Brown, C.G. *et al.* (2008) Accurate whole human genome sequencing using reversible terminator chemistry. *Nature*, **456**, 53–59.
11. Jasinska, A. and Krzyzosiak, W.J. (2004) Repetitive sequences that shape the human transcriptome. *FEBS Letters*, **567**, 136–141.
12. Waterston, R.H., Lindblad-Toh, K., Birney, E., Rogers, J., Abril, J.F., Agarwal, P. *et al.* (2002) Initial sequencing and comparative analysis of the mouse genome. *Nature*, **420**, 520–562.
13. Li, W.H., Gu, Z.L., Wang, H.D. and Nekrutenko, A. (2001) Evolutionary analyses of the human genome. *Nature*, **409**, 847–849.
14. Mikkelsen, T.S., Hillier, L.W., Eichler, E.E., Zody, M.C., Jaffe, D.B., Yang, S.P. *et al.* (2005) Initial sequence of the chimpanzee genome and comparison with the human genome. *Nature*, **437**, 69–87.
15. Britten, R.J. (2002) Divergence between samples of chimpanzee and human DNA sequences is 5%, counting indels. *Proceedings of the National Academy of Sciences of the United States of America*, **99**, 13633–13635.
16. Cann, R.L., Stoneking, M., Wilson, A.C. *et al.* (1987) Mitochondrial-DNA and human-evolution. *Nature*, **325**, 31–36.
17. Stringer, C.B. and Andrews, P. (1988) Genetic and fossil evidence for the origin of modern humans. *Science*, **239**, 1263–1268.
18. Sachidanandam, R., Weissman, D., Schmidt, S.C., Kakol, J.M., Stein, L.D., Marth, G. *et al.* (2001) A map of human genome sequence variation containing 1.42 million single nucleotide polymorphisms. *Nature*, **409**, 928–933.
19. Ahn, S.M., Kim, T.H., Lee, S., Kim, D., Ghang, H., Kim, D.S. *et al.* (2009) The first Korean genome sequence and analysis: full genome sequencing for a socio-ethnic group. *Genome Research*, **19**, 1622–1629.
20. Barbujani, G., Magagni, A., Minch, E. and CavalliSforza, L.L. (1997) An apportionment of human DNA diversity. *Proceedings of the National Academy of Sciences of the United States of America*, **94**, 4516–4519.
21. Lewontin, R.C. (1972) The apportionment of human diversity. *Evolutionary Biology*, **6**, 381–398.
22. Cavalli-Sforza, L.L., Menozzi, P. and Piazza, A. (1994) *The History and Geography of Human Genes*, Princeton University Press.
23. Serre, D. and Paabo, S.P. (2004) Evidence for gradients of human genetic diversity within and among continents. *Genome Research*, **14**, 1679–1685.

24. Handley, L.J.L., Manica, A., Goudet, J. and Balloux, F. (2007) Going the distance: human population genetics in a clinical world. *Trends in Genetics*, **23**, 432–439.
25. Abdulla, M.A., Ahmed, I., Assawamakin, A., Bhak, J., Brahmachari, S.K., Calacal, G.C. *et al.* (2009) Mapping human genetic diversity in Asia. *Science*, **326**, 1541–1545.
26. Lao, O., Lu, T.T., Nothnagel, M., Junge, O., Freitag-Wolf, S., Caliebe, A. *et al.* (2008) Correlation between genetic and geographic structure in Europe. *Current Biology*, **18**, 1241–1248.
27. Nelis, M., Esko. T., Magi, R., Zimprich, F., Zimprich, A., Toncheva, D. *et al.* (2009) Genetic structure of Europeans: a view from the north-east. *PLoS One*, **4**, e5472.
28. Jeffreys, A.J., Allen, M.J., Armour, J.A.L., Collick, A., Dubrova, Y., Fretwell, N. *et al.* (1995) Mutation processes at human minisatellites. *Electrophoresis*, **16**, 1577–1585.
29. Gill, P., Brinkmann, B., d'Ajola, E., Andersen, J., Bär, W., Carracedo, A., *et al.* (1997) Considerations from the European DNA profiling group (EDNAP) concerning STR nomenclature. *Forensic Science International*, **87**, 185–192.
30. Berg, I., Neumann, R., Cederberg, H., Rannug, U. and Jeffreys, A.J. (2003) Two modes of germline instability at human minisatellite MS1 (Locus D1S7): complex rearrangements and paradoxical hyperdeletion. *American Journal of Human Genetics*, **72**, 1436–1447.
31. Jeffreys, A.J., Wilson, V. and Thein, S.L. (1985) Hypervariable minisatellite regions in human DNA. *Nature*, **314**, 67–73.
32. Jeffreys, A.J., Brookfield, J.F.Y. and Semenoff, R. (1985) Positive identification of an immigration test-case using human DNA fingerprints. *Nature*, **317**, 818–819.
33. Gill, P., Jeffreys, A.J. and Werrett, D.J. (1985) Forensic application of DNA fingerprints. *Nature*, **318**, 577–579.
34. Thorisson, G.A. and Stein, L.D. (2003) The SNP Consortium website: past, present and future. *Nucleic Acids Research*, **31**, 124–127.
35. Gill, P. (2001) An assessment of the utility of single nucleotide polymorphisms (SNPs) for forensic purposes. *International Journal of Legal Medicine*, **114**, 204–210.
36. Krawczak, M. (1999) Informativity assessment for biallelic single nucleotide polymorphisms. *Electrophoresis*, **20**, 1676–1681.
37. Gill, P., Werrett, D.J., Budowle, B. and Guerrieri, R. (2004) An assessment of whether SNPs will replace STRs in national DNA databases. *Science and Justice*, **44**, 51–53.

3 Biological material – collection, characterization and storage

The sensitivity and evidential power of DNA profiling have impacted on the way in which crime scenes are investigated. Because only a few cells are required for DNA profiling, crime scene investigators now have a much wider range of biological evidence to collect and also have a much greater chance of contaminating the scene with their own DNA.

Sources of biological evidence

The human body is composed of trillions of cells and most of these contain a nucleus, mature red blood cells being a notable exception. A wide variety of cellular material can be recovered from crime scenes (Table 3.1).

Each nucleated cell contains two copies of an individual's genome and can be used, in theory, to generate a DNA profile under optimal conditions [1–3]. In practice, 15 or more cells are required to generate consistently good-quality DNA profiles from fresh material [4, 5]. Forensic samples usually show some level of degradation, and with higher levels of degradation, more cellular material is required to produce a DNA profile. If the material is very highly degraded then, even with the high sensitivity of DNA profiling, it may not be possible to generate a DNA profile.

The biological material encountered most often at scenes of crime is blood (Figure 3.1). This is mainly because of the violent nature of many crimes and also because it is easier to visualize than other biological fluids such as saliva.

Other frequently encountered samples include seminal fluid, which is of prime importance in sexual assault cases; saliva, which may be found on items either held in the mouth, such as cigarette butts and drinking vessels, or on bite marks, or in close proximity to the mouth when speaking, such as the inside of masks or phones; and epithelial cells, deposited, for example, as dandruff and in faeces. With the increase in the sensitivity of DNA profiling the recovery of DNA from epithelial cells shed on touching has also become possible [6]. Door handles, steering wheels and knife

An Introduction to Forensic Genetics Second Edition   William Goodwin, Adrian Linacre and Sibte Hadi
© 2011 John Wiley & Sons, Ltd

Table 3.1 Types of biological material that can be recovered from a crime scene. The DNA profiles generated from crime scene material are compared against reference profiles that are provided by suspects (or to a collection of reference samples held on a DNA database), and in some cases, the victims

Scenes of crime	Reference samples
Blood	Blood
Semen	Buccal swabs
Hair	Pulled hairs (containing roots)
Epithelial cells – shed skin cells:	
Saliva	–
Dandruff	–
Clothing	–
Cigarette butts	–
Drinking vessels/food	–
Urine	–
Vomit	–
Faeces	–
Touch DNA	–

(a)   (b)

Figure 3.1 Blood is the most common form of biological material that is recovered from crime scenes. (a) Large volumes of blood can be collected using a swab; if the blood is liquid then a syringe or pipette can be used. (Picture provided by Allan Scott, University of Central Lancashire.) (b) Blood on clothing is normally collected by swabbing or cutting out the stain. (Picture provided by Elizabeth Wilson)

handles are examples were no biological material is visible but is highly likely to be present. Hairs are naturally shed, and can also be pulled out through physical contact and can be recovered from crime scenes. Naturally shed hairs tend to have very little follicle attached and are not a good source of DNA, whereas plucked hairs or hairs removed because of a physical action often have the root attached, which is a rich source of cellular material.

The four most common nucleated cell types that are recovered from scenes of crime are white blood cells, spermatozoa, epithelial cells and hair follicles (Figure 3.2).

| (a) | (b) | (c) | (d) |

Figure 3.2 Common cell types that are recovered from scenes of crime: (a) white blood cells; (b) spermatozoa; (c) epithelial cells (from saliva); and (d) a hair shaft with the follicle attached. (The cells have been stained with haematoxylin and eosin)

Collection and handling of material at the crime scene

The high level of sensitivity that makes DNA profiling an invaluable forensic tool can also be a potential disadvantage. Contamination of evidential material with biological material from another source, such as an attending police officer or scene of crime officer, is a very real possibility. It is vital that the appropriate care is taken, such as maintaining the integrity of the scene and wearing full protective suits and face masks during the investigation of the scene [7–9] (Figure 3.3). Improper handling of the evidence can have serious consequences. In the worst cases, it can cause cross-contamination, lead to sample degradation and prevent or confuse the interpretation of evidence.

Identification and characterization of biological evidence

Locating biological material is necessary before collection for further analysis can occur. Furthermore, identification of the source of the material, for example demonstrating that a stain is blood, can be a vital piece of information in a given case, even before any DNA analysis is undertaken.

   Searching for biological material, both at the crime scene and in the forensic laboratory is performed primarily by eye. In the laboratory low-power search microscopes may help to localize stains and contact marks. The use of either chemical or physical methods can be used to detect biological materials. Alternative light sources (ALSs) using both infrared and ultraviolet light can provide a contrast between the fluorescence of proteins in the body fluid and the background substrate. Chemical methods use either the production of light or a colour change reaction. These techniques

Figure 3.3 It is standard practice for scene of crime officers to wear full overalls, shoe covers, gloves and face masks when collecting biological evidence from a scene of crime. Even with these precautions it is possible for crimes to be contaminated by forensic investigators, and it is becoming common for the DNA profiles of police officers and crime scene investigators to be stored on a database; any profiles recovered from the scene of crime can be checked against this elimination database to rule out the possibility of a profile coming from an investigating police or crime scene officer

have been developed to enable crime scene investigators and forensic biologists to utilize the inherent properties of biological evidence to both locate and characterize the material. When characterizing material there are two categories: presumptive and confirmatory. A range of presumptive and confirmatory tests is available that aids the identification of the three main body fluids encountered: blood, semen and saliva. Ideally, tests should be safe, inexpensive, simple to carry out, use a very small amount of the sample, be quick to perform and provide a simple indication of the presence or absence of a body fluid. The test should not affect the ability to carry out subsequent DNA profiling.

Presumptive tests can give false positives; however, in many circumstances, when the type of biological material is not of critical importance for a case, a positive result with a presumptive test will be sufficient information to move on to DNA analysis – which itself acts a confirmatory test for human biological material. In other circumstances, when the origin of the material is important, as is often the case with offences of a sexual nature, a confirmatory test is required that will unambiguously identify the biological material.

Blood

Blood is composed of liquid plasma, which contains soluble proteins, lipids, glucose, hormones, metabolites and salts, and the cellular component – red blood cells (erythrocytes), white blood cells (leucocytes) and platelets (thrombocytes).

Presumptive tests

In many cases blood will be clearly visible to the naked eye; however, if it is against a dark background or if the bloodstain has been cleaned, its detection may not be so straightforward. To help localize bloodstains an ALS, emitting at a wavelength of 415 nm light, will enhance bloodstains, which maximally absorb light at this wavelength and appear much darker than under white light [10, 11].

Searching a crime scene or items recovered from a crime scene for blood can also be aided by the use of luminol (3-amino-phthalhydrazide) dissolved in alkaline solution containing hydrogen peroxide or sodium perborate [12]. This solution can be sprayed on a wide area and will become oxidized and emit light by chemilumines-cence in the presence of haemoglobin and hydrogen peroxide (Figure 3.4) [13, 14]. It is necessary to be able to darken the area that is being searched in order that the chemiluminescence can be detected. Luminol can also be used in the more controlled environment of the forensic laboratory and can be particularly useful when searching clothing for trace amounts of blood. Fluorescein sprays can be used as an alternative to luminol: the detection levels are similar to luminol, but it has the advantage that it can be used in lighter environments, although an alternative light source, at 450 nm, is required for detection [15]. In both cases, the presence of haemoglobin produces a light blue light that fades after approximately 30 seconds. A solution can be reapplied and the fluorescence activated a couple of times until the haemoglobin is saturated.

Other presumptive tests are available that, like luminol and fluorescein, take advantage of the peroxidase-like activity of the haem group, which is abundant as part of the haemoglobin molecule within red blood cells. The haem catalyses the hydrolysis of hydrogen peroxide, which in turn leads to the oxidation of the target chemical compound, resulting in a colour change. Commonly used chemi-cal compounds include leucomalachite green (LMG) (colourless to blue-green) [13],

Figure 3.4 Luminol, sprayed onto recovered objects or at the crime scene, gives out a blue fluorescence on contact with blood; a limitation is that the test has to be carried out in a dark conditions. The detection of potential bloodstains using this method requires further confirmatory analysis to avoid false positives

(a)   (b)   (c)

Figure 3.5 In the presence of haem and hydrogen peroxide the chemical colour change can be seen. To perform a Kastle–Mayer (KM) test a piece of filter paper is folded in half and then half again to make a corner (b). This is rubbed gently against the blood, transferring a trace of the dried stain to the filter paper. A drop of KM solution (should give no change by itself) followed by a drop of H_2O_2 leads to a pink/purple colour reaction in the presence of haemoglobin (c)

phenolphthalein (Kastle–Meyer reagent) (colourless to pink) and tetramethylbenzidine (TMB) (colourless to green) [16–19] (Figure 3.5).

Any biological material that contains peroxidase activity, such as some plant extracts, or any material that leads to the hydrolysis of hydrogen peroxide can also result in a false positive [20, 21].

Confirmatory tests

The Teichman and Takayama crystal tests, which are based on the formation of haem-derived crystals, were developed in 1853 and 1912, respectively [17], but, along with other microscopic and spectroscopic techniques, are rarely used now [22]. Two relatively new confirmatory tests offer some advantages over previous tests: messenger RNA (mRNA) analysis allows the origins of several different types of biological material to be identified; and flow immunochromatographic strip tests offer a simple and sensitive test for human blood.

mRNA expression analysis has been shown to be a viable confirmatory test [23–27], even in bloodstains that are several months old [28]. The targets that are amplified are blood-specific, such as the β-spectrin (SPTB) [23, 25, 27], porphobilinogen deaminase (PBGD) [27], δ-aminolevulinate synthase (ALAS2) [25] and the alpha locus 1 (HBA) marker [29]; the methodology can also be used to differentiate between menstrual and vascular blood, targeting the menstrual blood-specific matrix metalloproteinase-7 (MMP-7) transcript [24, 30, 31]. The major drawback of mRNA technology is that it requires specialist techniques and is a more complex process than DNA profiling itself; however, the extra probative value of identifying the origin of the blood will be very valuable in some cases.

An antibody-based lateral flow immunochromatographic strip test is relatively easy to perform. The test involves reacting the suspected bloodstain with a glycophorin A antibody (glycophorin A is found in the membranes of red blood cells). The mixture is applied to and migrates along a membrane; if blood is present a visible complex is formed with an immobilized capture antibody (Figure 3.6) [32].

Figure 3.6 The lateral flow immunology test shows two bands in a positive test whereas in a negative test only one band is present. Positive tests are shown from left to right for blood, semen, saliva. A test is also available for urine

Semen

Semen comprises mature sperm (spermatozoa) suspended in a fluid secreted from the prostate gland, seminal vesicles, Cowper's gland and the glands of Littré [16]. The positive identification of semen can be extremely important evidence to support an allegation of sexual assault and both presumptive and definitive tests are commonly used.

Presumptive tests

As with blood, ALS can be a powerful technique to locate and presumptively identify semen. Semen produces strong photoluminescence over a range of wavelengths – exposed to UV light it will emit blue photoluminescence that will be visible to the naked eye [10, 11, 33]; as with other ALS-based methods false positives are detected [11, 33, 34].

A simple, and commonly used, test involves assaying for the presence of the enzyme seminal acid phosphatase (SAP), which is present in high concentrations in seminal fluid [16]. Other body fluids, such as saliva and vaginal secretions, contain the enzyme albeit in significantly lower concentrations and so can give a positive result [35]. The presence of SAP is tested for by its ability to catalyse the hydrolysis of organic phosphate, for example α-naphthyl phosphate, which following hydrolysis will react with Brentamine Fast Blue (a diazonium salt chromogen), leading to a colour change [22]. Other biological material containing acid phosphatases can lead to false positives, such as plant material and vaginal secretions, although the reaction with semen is usually stronger, and therefore the colour change faster, than with other material. SAP is quick, simple and safe to perform. As it is an enzyme-based test, old stains may give a slower reaction, and therefore a longer colour change, and in some case no reaction may occur if the enzyme no longer functions.

Confirmatory tests

The most commonly used confirmatory test for semen is visualization of the spermatozoa following staining; commonly used dyes are haematoxylin and eosin (Figure 3.2b) and Christmas tree stain, which stains heads red and tails green [36].

Another marker for the identification of semen is the protein P30, which is a prostate-specific antigen (PSA) [37, 38]. The advantage of using PSA compared with the reaction involving acid phosphatase is that PSA is produced independently from the generation of sperm and therefore it can be used for both spermic and azoospermic samples; it is also very sensitive and resistant to degradation, even in cadavers [39]. Detection of PSA is most common with the use of the immunochromatographic strip test, using antibodies raised against human PSA [40–42] (Figure 3.6).

Another confirmatory test is mRNA analysis, detecting the semen-specific protamine (PRM)1, PRM2 and kallikrein 3 (PSA) genes [24, 28, 29].

Saliva

Saliva is a fluid produced in the mouth to aid in swallowing and the initial stage of digestion. A healthy person produces between 1 L and 1.5 L of saliva every day and can transfer saliva, along with epithelial cells sloughed off from the buccal cavity, in a number of ways. Transfer may be by contact, such as on food products when eating, drinking vessels, cigarette butts, envelopes or in oral sexual assaults. Transfer may also be by aerial deposition of saliva such as on to the front of a mask when worn over the head or on to a telephone when talking into the mouthpiece.

Presumptive tests

As with blood and semen ALS can be used to locate saliva; stains appear blue-white when viewed under UV light. Most presumptive tests for saliva make use of the enzyme α-amylase, which is present at high concentrations and digests starch and complex sugars. The α-amylase enzyme hydrolyses $\alpha1–4$ glycosidic bonds in glucose polymers, such as glycogen and starch. The digestion of starch can be assessed using the starch–iodine test: a sample of the evidential stain is incubated with a starch solution; iodine is then added and if the starch has been broken down the solution will be clear, whereas if starch is still present the colour will be blue. The technique is not widely used as more sensitive assays have been developed using modified starch that is covalently linked to a dye, such as cibachron blue or procion red, to form an insoluble complex [43–45]; in the presence of α-amylase activity the dye is released from the complex and becomes soluble. The release of the dye causes a colour change that can easily be detected, either in solution or by its ability to migrate through an otherwise impermeable barrier, such as paper [43–45] (Figure 3.7). Amylases are present in other body fluids such as sweat, vaginal fluid, breastmilk and pancreatic secretions; however, amylase is present in saliva at concentrations greater than in other body fluids [44, 46]. The process takes at least 30 minutes to complete and, unlike the tests for blood and SAP for semen, can only be performed in the laboratory. The test for saliva is only used in specific tests, such as oral sexual assault cases.

Confirmatory tests

Until recently there were no readily used confirmatory tests for saliva. As with blood and semen, antibody tests, using lateral flow strips, have been developed that are specific for saliva [47–49]. mRNA can also be isolated from saliva; detection of several transcripts can provide confirmation that a stain contains saliva [23, 24, 50, 51].

Epithelial cells

When an object is touched, epithelial cells may be deposited [6]. The amount of cellular material transferred depends upon the amount of time the skin is in contact with the object, the amount of pressure applied, and the presence of fluid such as sweat to mediate the transfer. Some people transfer their skin cells more readily than others; these people are classified as good shedders [9]. This material can be collected from evidential material by swabbing or by tape lifting [52, 53]. Surfaces that the perpetrator(s) of a crime are likely to have had contact with include door handles, the ends of ligatures [54], the handles of weapons and contact marks on victims. These are all potential sources of epithelial cells [55]. In most cases the number of cells is very low and the success rate of DNA profiling is limited. Screening methods, for example using the reagent ninhydrin, which detects the presence of amino acids (and is routinely used to develop latent fingerprints), can be helpful in identifying samples that are likely to contain epithelial cells [56]. Epithelial cells, as with saliva and semen stains, may fluoresce at different wavelengths of light compared with the background substrate and can be enhanced under some conditions [10, 11, 57].

Evidence collection

The success in finding biological material depends upon the search method employed and also on the integrity and state of the scene. In the UK, biological material is

(a)

(b)

(c)

Figure 3.7 Location of saliva using Phadebas® paper. (a) Even with appropriate lighting the identification of saliva stains can be difficult. (b) The article being examined is moistened using sterile DNA-free water and Phadebas® paper is placed on top with the carbohydrate dye-coated side in contact with the fabric; a glass plate holds the paper in contact. (c) α-amylase breaks down the carbohydrate-dye complex, and the dye migrates through the paper and can be visualized found at approximately 12% of investigated crime scenes; this figure can go up significantly if the crime scene is exhaustively searched [58].

The methods used for collection will vary depending on the type of sample. Dry stains and contact marks on large immovable items are normally collected using a sterile swab that has been moistened with distilled water [59, 60]; in other cases, scraping or cutting of material may be more appropriate. Lifting from the surface using high-quality adhesive tape is an alternative method for collecting epithelial cells [52]. Liquid blood can be collected using a syringe or pipette and transferred to a clean sterile storage tube that contains anticoagulant (ethylene-diamine tetraacetic acid (EDTA)), or by using a swab or piece of fabric to soak up the stain, which should be air dried to prevent the build up of microbial activity [8]. Liquid blood can also be applied to FTA® paper, which is impregnated with chemicals to prevent the action of microbial agents and stabilize the DNA. (FTA® paper was developed by *Flinders* Technology Associates.)

Smaller movable objects, such as weapons, which might contain biological material are packaged at the scene of crime and examined in the controlled environment of the forensic laboratory. The same range of swabbing, scraping and lifting techniques as used in the field can be employed to collect the biological material. Clothing taken from suspects and victims presents an important source of biological evidence. This is also analysed in the forensic biology laboratory, where stains and contact areas can be recorded and then cut out or swabbed.

Sexual and physical assault

Following sexual assaults, the victim should be examined as soon after the event as possible. Semen is recovered by a trained medical examiner using standard swabs; fingernail scrapings can be collected using a variety of swabs; combings of pubic and head hair are normally stored in paper envelopes. The samples collected by the medical examiner are dependent on the nature of the allegation and information given by the alleged victim. Contact marks, for example bruising caused by gripping or bite marks, can be swabbed for DNA. The same types of evidence (except semen) can be taken after cases of physical assault [8].

Reference samples

In order to identify samples recovered from the scene of crime, reference samples are needed for comparison. Reference samples are provided by a suspect and, in some cases, a victim. Traditionally, blood samples have been taken and these provide an abundant supply of DNA; however, they are invasive and blood samples are a potential health hazard. Buccal swabs that are rubbed on the inner surface of the cheek to collect cellular material have replaced blood samples in many scenarios. In some circumstances plucked hairs may be used, but this source of material is not commonly used.

Figure 3.8 FTA® cards can be used to store both blood and buccal cells. The cellular material lyses on contact with the card. The DNA binds to the card and is stable for years at room temperature

FTA® cards can be used to store both buccal and blood samples (Figure 3.8). The FTA® card is a cellulose-based paper which is impregnated with chemicals that cause cellular material to break open; the DNA is released and binds to the card. The chemicals on the card also inhibit any bacterial or fungal growth and DNA can be stably stored on FTA® cards for years at room temperature as long as the card remains dry.

Storage of biological material

Biological material collected for DNA analysis should be stored in conditions that will slow the rate of DNA degradation, in particular low temperatures and low humidity. A cool and dry environment limits the action of bacteria and fungi that find biological material a rich source of food and can rapidly degrade biological material.

The exact conditions depend on the nature of the samples and the environment in which the samples are to be stored. Buccal swabs and swabs used to collect material at a crime scene can be stored under refrigeration for short periods and are either frozen directly or dried and then stored at $-20\,^{\circ}$C for longer term storage. Blood samples will normally be stored at between $-20\,^{\circ}$C and $-80\,^{\circ}$C. Buccal and blood samples collected using FTA® cards can be stored for years at room temperature. Some items of evidence, like clothing, can be stored in a cool dry room; in temperate regions of the world DNA has been recovered from material stored at room temperature for several years [59]. When samples are not frozen, for example clothing, they are stored in acid-free paper rather than plastic bags, to minimize the build up of any moisture. Once the DNA has been extracted from a sample, the DNA can be stored short term at $4\,^{\circ}$C but should be stored at $-20\,^{\circ}$C to $-80\,^{\circ}$C for long-term storage.

References

1. Kloosterman, A.D. and Kersbergen, P. (2003) Efficacy and limits of genotyping low copy number DNA samples by multiplex PCR of STR loci. *Progress in Forensic Genetics*, **9**, 795–798.

2. Li, H.H., Cui, X.F. and Arnheim, N. (1990) Direct electrophoretic detection of the allelic state of single DNA-molecules in human sperm by using the polymerase chain-reaction. *Proceedings of the National Academy of Sciences of the United States of America*, **87**, 4580–4584.

3. Li, H.H., Gyllensten, U.B., Cui, X.F., Saiki, R.K., Erlich, H.A. and Arnheim, N. (1988) Amplification and analysis of DNA-sequences in single human-sperm and diploid-cells. *Nature*, **335**, 414–417.

4. Gill, P. (2001) Application of low copy number DNA profiling. *Croatian Medical Journal*, **42**, 229–232.

5. Gill, P., Whitaker, J., Flaxman, C., Brown, N. and Buckleton, J. (2000) An investigation of the rigor of interpretation rules for STRs derived from less than 100 pg of DNA. *Forensic Science International*, **112**, 17–40.

6. van Oorschot, R.A.H. and Jones, M.K. (1997) DNA fingerprints from fingerprints. *Nature*, **387**, 767–767.

7. Lee, H.C. and Ladd, C. (2001) Preservation and collection of biological evidence. *Croation Medical Journal*, **42**, 225–228.

8. Lee, H.C., Ladd, C., Scherczinger, C.A. and Bourke, M.T. (1998) Forensic applications of DNA typing part 2: collection and preservation of DNA evidence. *American Journal of Forensic Medicine and Pathology*, **19**, 10–18.

9. Rutty, G.N., Hopwood, A. and Tucker, V. (2003) The effectiveness of protective clothing in the reduction of potential DNA contamination of the scene of crime. *International Journal of Legal Medicine*, **117**, 170–174.

10. Stoilovic, M. (1991) Detection of semen and blood stains using polilight as a light-source. *Forensic Science International*, **51**, 289–296.

11. Vandenberg, N. and Oorschot, R.A.H. (2006) The use of Polilight((R)) in the detection of seminal fluid, saliva, and bloodstains and comparison with conventional chemical-based screening tests. *Journal of Forensic Sciences*, **51**, 361–370.

12. Quickenden, T.I. and Cooper, P.D. (2001) Increasing the specificity of the forensic luminol test for blood. *Luminescence*, **16**, 251–253.

13. Grodsky, M., Wright, K. and Kirk, P.L. (1951) Simplified preliminary blood testing: an improved technique and a comparative study of methods. *Journal of Criminal Law and Criminology and Police Science*, **42**, 95–104.

14. Sprecht, W. (1937) Chemiluminesenz des hamins, ein hilfsmittel zur auffindung und erkennung forensisch wichturger blutspuren. *Angewandte Chemie*, **1937**, 155–157.

15. Budowle, B., Leggitt, J.L., Defenbaugh, D.A., Keys. K.M. and Malkiewicz, S.F. (2000) The presumptive reagent fluorescein for detection of dilute bloodstains and subsequent STR typing of recovered DNA. *Journal of Forensic Sciences*, **45**, 1090–1092.

16. Ballantyne, J. (2000) Serology, in *Encyclopedia of Forensic Sciences* (eds J.A. Siegel *et al.*), Academic Press, pp. 1322–1331.

17. Lee, H. and Pagliaro, E. (2000) Blood Identification, in *Encyclopedia of Forensic Sciences* (eds J.A. Siegel *et al.*), Academic Press, pp. 1331–1338.

18. Hunt, A.C., Corby, C. and Dodd, B.E. (1960) The identification of human stains – a critical survey. *Journal of Forensic Medicine*, **7**, 112–130.

19. Poon, H., Elliott, J., Modler, J. and Fregeau, C. (2009) The use of hemastix (R) and the subsequent lack of DNA recovery using the promega DNA IQ (TM) system. *Journal of Forensic Sciences*, **54**, 1278–1286.

20. Tobe, S.S., Watson, N. and Nic Daeid, N. (2007) Evaluation of six presumptive tests for blood, their specificity, sensitivity, and effect on high molecular-weight DNA. *Journal of Forensic Sciences*, **52**, 102–109.

21. Quickenden, T.I. and Creamer, J.I. (2001) A study of common interferences with the forensic luminol test for blood. *Luminescence*, **16**, 295–298.

22. Virkler, K. and Lednev, I.K. (2009) Analysis of body fluids for forensic purposes: from laboratory testing to non-destructive rapid confirmatory identification at a crime scene. *Forensic Science International*, **188**, 1–17.

23. Alvarez, M., Juusola, J. and Ballantyne, J. (2004) An mRNA and DNA co-isolation method for forensic casework samples. *Analytical Biochemistry*, **335**, 289–298.

24. Juusola, J. and Ballantyne, J. (2005) Multiplex mRNA profiling for the identification of body fluids. *Forensic Science International*, **152**, 1–12.
25. Juusola, J. and Ballantyne, J. (2007) mRNA profiling for body fluid identification by multiplex quantitative RT-PCR. *Journal of Forensic Sciences*, **52**, 1252–1262.
26. Setzer, M., Juusola, J and Ballantyne, J. (2008) Recovery and stability of RNA in vaginal swabs and blood, semen, and saliva stains. *Journal of Forensic Sciences*, **53**, 296–305.
27. Juusola, J. and Ballantyne, J. (2003) Messenger RNA profiling: a prototype method to supplant conventional methods for body fluid identification. *Forensic Science International*, **135**, 85–96.
28. Haas, C., Klesser, B., Maake, C., Bar, W. and Kratzer, A. (2009) rnRNA profiling for body fluid identification by reverse transcription endpoint PCR and realtime PCR. *Forensic Science International: Genetics*, **3**, 80–88.
29. Nussbaumer, C., Gharehbaghi-Schnell, E. and Korschineck, I. (2006) Messenger RNA profiling: a novel method for body fluid identification by Real-Time PCR. *Forensic Science International*, **157**, 181–186.
30. Bauer, M. and Patzelt, D. (2002) Evaluation of mRNA markers for the identification of menstrual blood. *Journal of Forensic Sciences*, **47**, 1278–1282.
31. Bauer, M. and Patzelt, D. (2008) Identification of menstrual blood by real time RT-PCR: technical improvements and the practical value of negative test results. *Forensic Science International*, **174**, 54–58.
32. (2008) Independent Forensics Rapid Stain Identification of human blood (RSID™-Blood), technical information sheet.
33. Santucci, K.A., Nelson, D.G., McQuillen, K.K., Duffy, S.J. and Linakis, J.G. (1999) Wood's lamp utility in the identification of semen. *Pediatrics*, **104**, 1342–1344.
34. Nelson, D.G. and Santucci, K.A. (2002) An alternate light source to detect semen. *Academic Emergency Medicine*, **9**, 1045–1048.
35. Steinman, G. (1995) Rapid spot tests for identifying suspected semen specimens. *Forensic Science International*, **72**, 191–197.
36. Allery, J.P., Telmon, N., Mieusset, R., Blanc, A. and Rouge, D. (2001) Cytological detection of spermatozoa: comparison of three staining methods. *Journal of Forensic Sciences*, **46**, 349–351.
37. Graves, H.C.B., Sensabaugh, G.F. and Blake, E.T. (1985) Postcoital detection of a male-specific semen protein – application to the investigation of rape. *New England Journal of Medicine*, **312**, 338–343.
38. Simich, J.P., Morris, S.L., Klick, R.L. and Rittenhouse-Diakun, K. (1999) Validation of the use of a commercially available kit for the identification of prostate specific antigen (PSA) in semen stains. *Journal of Forensic Sciences*, **44**, 1229–1231.
39. Healy, D.A., Hayes, C.J., Leonard, P., McKenna, L. and O'Kennedy, R. (2007) Biosensor developments: application to prostate-specific antigen detection. *Trends in Biotechnology*, **25**, 125–131.
40. Maher, J., Vintiner, S., Elliot, D. and Melia, L. (2002) Evaluation of the BioSign (TM) PSA membrane test for the identification of semen stains in forensic casework. *New Zealand Medical Journal*, **115**, 48–49.
41. Hochmeister, M.N., Budowle, B., Rudin, O., Gehrig, C., Borer, U., Thali, M. *et al.* (1999) Evaluation of prostate-specific antigen (PSA) membrane test assays for the forensic identification of seminal fluid. *Journal of Forensic Sciences*, **44**, 1057–1060.
42. Pang, B.C.M. and Cheung, B.K.K. (2007) Identification of human semenogelin in membrane strip test as an alternative method for the detection of semen. *Forensic Science International*, **169**, 27–31.
43. Willott, G.M. and Griffiths, M. (1980) New method for locating saliva stains – spotty paper for spotting spit. *Forensic Science International*, **15**, 79–83.
44. Martin, N.C., Clayson, N.J. and Scrimger, D.G. (2006) The sensitivity and specificity of Red-Starch paper for the detection of saliva. *Science and Justice*, **46**, 97–105.
45. Whitehead, P.H. and Kipps, A.E. (1975) Test paper for detecting saliva stains. *Journal of the Forensic Science Society*, **15**, 39–42.

46. Auvdel, M.J. (1986) Amylase levels in semen and saliva stains. *Journal of Forensic Sciences*, **31**, 426–431.
47. Casey, D.G. and Price, J. (2010) The sensitivity and specificity of the RSID (TM)-saliva kit for the detection of human salivary amylase in the Forensic Science Laboratory, Dublin, Ireland. *Forensic Science International*, **194**, 67–71.
48. Old, J.B., Schweers, B.A., Boonlayangoor, P.W. and Reich, K.A. (2009) Developmental validation of RSID (TM)-saliva: a lateral flow immunochromatographic strip test for the forensic detection of saliva. *Journal of Forensic Sciences*, **54**, 866–873.
49. Pang, B.C.M. and Cheung, B.K.K. (2008) Applicability of two commercially available kits for forensic identification of saliva stains. *Journal of Forensic Sciences*, **53**, 1117–1122.
50. Zubakov, D., Hanekamp, E., Kokshoorn, M., van Ijcken, W., Kayser, M. (2008) Stable RNA markers for identification of blood and saliva stains revealed from whole genome expression analysis of time-wise degraded samples. *International Journal of Legal Medicine*, **122**, 135–142.
51. Zubakov, D., Kokshoorn, M., Kloosterman, A. and Kayser, M. (2009) New markers for old stains: stable mRNA markers for blood and saliva identification from up to 16-year-old stains. *International Journal of Legal Medicine*, **123**, 71–74.
52. Hall, D. and Fairley, M. (2004) A single approach to the recovery of DNA and firearm discharge residue evidence. *Science and Justice*, **44**, 15–19.
53. van Oorschot, R.A.H., Phelan, D.G., Furlong, S., Scarfo, G.M., Holding, N.L. and Cummins, M.J. (2003) Are you collecting all the available DNA from touched objects? *Progress in Forensic Genetics*, **9**, 803–807.
54. Bohnert, M., Faller-Marquardt, M., Lutz, S., Amberg, R., Weisser, H.J. and Pollak, S. (2001) Transfer of biological traces in cases of hanging and ligature strangulation. *Forensic Science International*, **116**, 107–115.
55. Wiegand, P. and Kleiber, M. (1997) DNA typing of epithelial cells after strangulation. *International Journal of Legal Medicine*, **110**, 181–183.
56. Anslinger, K., Selbertinger, U., Bayer, B., Rolf, B. and Eisenmenger, W. (2004) Ninhydrin treatment as a screening method for the suitability of swabs taken from contact stains for DNA analysis. *International Journal of Legal Medicine*, **118**, 122–124.
57. Soukos, N.S., Crowley, K., Bamberg, M.P., Gillies, R., Doukas, A.G. and Evans, R. (2000) A rapid method to detect dried saliva stains swabbed from human skin using fluorescence spectroscopy. *Forensic Science International*, **114**, 133–138.
58. National Policing Improvement Agency (2009) National DNA Database annual report 2007–2009.
59. Benecke, M. (2005) Forensic DNA samples – collection and handling, in *Encyclopedia of medical Genomics and Proteomics* (eds J. Fuchs and M. Podda), Marcel Dekker, pp. 500–504.
60. Sweet, D., Lorente, M., Lorente, J.A., Valenzuela, A. and Villanueva, E. (1997) An improved method to recover saliva from human skin: The double swab technique. *Journal of Forensic Sciences*, **42**, 320–322.

4 DNA extraction and quantification

DNA extraction has two main aims: first, to maximizing the yield of DNA from a sample and in sufficient quantity to permit a full DNA profile to be obtained – this is increasingly important as the sample size diminishes; and, second, to extract DNA that is pure enough for subsequent analysis: the level of difficulty here depends very much on the nature of the sample. Once the DNA has been extracted, quantifying the DNA is important for subsequent analysis.

DNA extraction

There are many methods available for extracting DNA. The choice of which method to use depends on a number of factors, including the sample type and quantity; the speed and in some cases ability to automate the extraction procedure [1–5]; the success rate with forensic samples, which is a result of extracting the maximum amount of DNA from a sample and at the same time removing any PCR inhibitors that will prevent successful profiling [2, 6–8]; the chemicals that are used in the extraction – most laboratories go to great lengths to avoid using hazardous chemicals; and the cost of the procedure. Another important factor is the experience of the laboratory staff.

General principles of DNA extraction

The three stages of DNA extraction can be classified as (i) disruption of the cellular membranes, resulting in cell lysis, (ii) protein denaturation and (iii) the separation of DNA from the denatured protein and other cellular components. Some of the extraction methods commonly used in forensic laboratories are described below.

Chelex® 100 resin

The Chelex® 100 method was one of the first extraction techniques adopted by the forensic community. Chelex® 100 is a resin that is composed of styrene–divinylbenzene copolymers containing paired iminodiacetate ions [9]. The resin

An Introduction to Forensic Genetics Second Edition   William Goodwin, Adrian Linacre and Sibte Hadi

Figure 4.1 The Chelex® 100 extraction is quick and easy to perform. (a) The cellular material is added to 1 ml of TE (1 mm EDTA, 10 mm Tris: pH 8.0) and incubated at room temperature for 10–15 minutes. (b) The tube is centrifuged at high speed to pellet the cellular material and the supernatant is removed. (c) The pellet of cellular material is resuspended in 5% Chelex®, the tube is incubated at 56 °C for 15–30 minutes and then placed in a boiling water bath for 8 minutes. The tube is centrifuged at high speed for 2–3 minutes to pellet precipitated protein. (d) The supernatant contains the DNA and can be used directly in a PCR

has a very high affinity for polyvalent metal ions, such as magnesium (Mg^{2+}); it chelates the polyvalent metal ions and effectively removes them from solution. The extraction procedure is very simple, the Chelex® 100 resin, which is supplied as beads, is made into a 5% suspension using distilled water. The cellular material is incubated with the Chelex® 100 suspension at 56 °C for up to 30 minutes. Proteinase K, which digests most cellular protein, is often added at this point. This incubation is followed by 8–10 minutes at 100 °C to ensure that all the cells have ruptured and that the protein has denatured. The tube is then simply centrifuged to pellet the Chelex® 100 resin and the denatured protein at the bottom of the tube, leaving the aqueous solution containing the DNA to be used in PCR (Figure 4.1). The Chelex® 100 suspension is alkaline, between pH 9.0 and 11.0, and as a result DNA that is isolated using this procedure is single-stranded.

The major advantages of this method are it is quick, taking around a hour; it is simple and does not involve the movement of liquid between tubes, thereby reducing the possibility of accidentally mixing samples; the cost is very low; and it avoids the use of harmful chemicals. Importantly, it is amenable to a wide range of forensic samples [9]. The DNA extract produced using this method is relatively crude but sufficiently clean in most cases to generate a DNA profile.

Silica-based DNA extraction

Within molecular biology generally, the 'salting out' procedure has been widely used [1]. The first stage of the extraction involves incubating the cellular material in a lysis buffer that contains a detergent along with proteinase K. The commonly used detergents are sodium dodecyl sulphate (SDS), Tween 20, Triton X-100 and

Nonidet P-40. The lysis buffer destabilizes the cell membranes, leading to the break-down of cellular structure.

The addition of a chaotropic salt, for example 6 M guanidine thiocyanate [10] or 6 M sodium chloride, during or after cell lysis, disrupts the protein structure by interfering with hydrogen bonding, Van der Waals interactions and hydrophobic interactions. Cellular proteins are largely insoluble in the presence of the chaotropic agent and can be removed by centrifugation or filtration. The reduced solubility of the cellular protein is caused by the excess of ions in the high concentration of salt competing with the proteins for the aqueous solvent, effectively dehydrating the protein. Commonly used commercial kits, for example the Qiagen kits, exploit the salting-out procedure; the methods to isolate the DNA after the cellular disruption vary widely.

Several DNA extraction methods are based on the binding properties of silica or glass particles. DNA will bind to silica or glass particles with a high affinity in the presence of a chaotropic salt [10, 11]. After the other cellular components have been removed the DNA can be released from the silica/glass particles by suspending them in water (Figure 4.2). In the absence of the chaotropic salt the DNA no longer binds to the silica/glass and is released into solution. The silica method, in particular, has been shown to be robust when extracting DNA from forensic samples [2]; it is also amenable to automation [2–4].

The advantage of the silica-based salting-out methods are that they yield high molecular weight DNA that is cleaner than DNA from Chelex® 100 extractions. As with Chelex® 100 extractions, no highly toxic chemicals are involved. The process takes longer than the Chelex® 100 and involves more than one change of tube and so increases the possibility of sample mixing and cross-contamination.

Phenol–chloroform-based DNA extraction

The phenol–chloroform method has been widely used in molecular biology but has been slowly phased out since the mid-1990s, largely because of the toxic nature of phenol. It is still used in some forensic laboratories; in particular, it is still widely used for the extraction of DNA from bone samples and soils.

Cell lysis is performed as in the previous method. Phenol–chloroform is added to the cell lysate and mixed – the phenol denatures the protein. The extract is then centrifuged and the precipitated protein forms a pellicle at the interface between the organic phenol–chloroform phase and the aqueous phase; this process is repeated two to three times or until there is no visible pellicle [12]. The DNA is then purified from the aqueous phase by ethanol precipitation or filter centrifugation (Figure 4.3). The method produces clean DNA but has some drawbacks: in addition to the toxic nature of phenol, multiple tube changes are required and the process is labour intensive.

FTA paper

In Chapter 3 FTA® paper was described as a method for sample collection and storage, particularly from buccal swabs and fresh blood samples. Once a sample is

Figure 4.2 DNA extraction from buccal cells using a salting-out method based on the QIAamp® Blood Mini Kit. (a) Cellular material is added to a lysis buffer and proteinase K and incubated at 56 °C for at least 15 minutes. (b) Ethanol is added to the solution before it is transferred in order to provide the optimum DNA binding conditions. (c) The lysis solution is then transferred to a spin basket that has a membrane that will bind the DNA in the presence of the chaotropic salt. (d) The spin basket is centrifuged and the DNA is captured by the membrane as the solution passes through. (e) Wash buffers are added to the spin basket and (f) pass through the membrane when centrifuged. (g) Typically 100 μl of elution buffer is added to the membrane; in the absence of the chaotropic salt the DNA is released from the membrane and (h) is recovered upon a final centrifugation

applied to the FTA® paper it is stable at room temperature for several years. Cellular material lyses on contact with the FTA® paper and the DNA becomes bound to the paper, which has been treated with chemicals to inhibit the growth of microorganisms that might otherwise break down the DNA.

To analyse the DNA sample, the first step is to take a small region of the card, normally a 2 mm diameter circle, place it into a 1.5 ml tube and the non-DNA components are simply washed off, leaving only DNA on the card. The small circle of FTA® paper is then added directly to a PCR (Figure 4.4). The FTA® paper

Figure 4.3 DNA extraction from a buccal swab cells using a salting-out method based on phenol-chloroform. (a) Cellular material is added to a lysis buffer and proteinase K and incubated at 56 °C for at least 15 minutes. (b and c) The swab is removed and phenol is added, the solution is then vortexed and centrifuged. Precipitated protein and carbohydrate form a pellicle at the interface; this step is repeated until there is no visible material at the interface. Protocols vary – some use only phenol, others phenol and chloroform (isoamyl alcohol may be added to the phenol/chloroform mixture to prevent it separating). (d) In a final step chloroform alone is added; this removes any residual phenol, which would inhibit downstream processes such as PCR. The aqueous phase now contains DNA. This can be concentrated by adding sodium acetate and either ethanol or iso-propanol to precipitate the DNA, followed by centrifugation (the DNA will precipitate and form a pellet) or by using filter centrifugation, which is similar to the steps in Figure 4.2g–f, except that the membrane acts as a molecular sieve – allowing small molecules to pass through while retaining DNA strands

extractions are very simple to perform and do not require multiple tube changes, thus reducing the possibility of sample mixing [13–19]. The technology also provides a simple and relatively inexpensive method for long-term storage of DNA, removing the requirement for refrigeration.

DNA extraction from challenging samples

The extraction of the many samples encountered in the forensic laboratory, including blood and shed epithelial cells, can be carried out routinely using any of the above techniques. There are however some sample types that necessitate variations on the basic techniques.

Semen

Semen is one of the most commonly encountered types of biological evidence. The extraction of DNA from the spermatozoa is complicated by the structure of the spermatozoa (Figure 4.5). DNA is found within the head of the spermatozoa that

Figure 4.4   DNA extraction from blood on FTA® paper. (a) Sections of the FTA® card are removed with a punch (usually 1.2 mm or 2 mm diameter), added to FTA® purification reagent, mixed and incubated at room temperature for 5 minutes; one or more punched discs can be added to the extraction. (b) The liquid is removed and replaced with fresh purification reagent; this process is repeated two or three times. (c) The discs are then washed two or three times in TE (10 mm Tris-HCl, 0.1 mm EDTA, pH 8.0). (d) Finally, the TE is removed and the FTA® discs, containing the DNA, are left to dry at room temperature or with gentle heat (approximately 50 °C). The discs can now be added directly to a PCR reaction

Figure 4.5   The nucleus in the spermatozoa is protected by the acrosome

is capped by the protective acrosome, which is rich in the amino acid cysteine; a large number of disulfide bridges form between the cysteine residues in the acrosome. Proteinase K, which is a general proteinase, cannot break the disulfide bonds: however, the addition of dithiothreitol (DTT), a reducing agent that will break the disulfide bonds, greatly increases the release of spermatozoa DNA [20].

Another complication with semen is that it is often recovered as a mixture of spermatozoa and epithelial cells. The acrosome can be an advantage in these cases as it is possible to perform differential lysis: the epithelial cells are broken down by mild lysis conditions and the spermatozoa can be effectively separated from the lysed epithelial cells [20, 21].

Hair shafts

Hair shafts that have been pulled out often possess a root that is rich in cellular material and DNA can be extracted using any of the commonly used techniques – plucked roots have been shown to contain as much as 0.5 µg of DNA [22]. Hair that has been shed when it is in the resting telogen phase often contains no cellular material around the root. The hair shafts are composed of keratin, trace metals, air and pigment – cell fragments, including DNA can get trapped in the matrix of the hair and provide enough DNA to produce a profile. However, hair is notoriously difficult to analyse, and in many cases it is only possible to successfully profile mitochondrial DNA [22], although nuclear DNA can, in some cases, be recovered [23].

The hair shaft, like the spermatozoa acrosome, is rich in disulfide bridges and requires either mechanical grinding [24] or the addition of a reducing agent such as DTT [22, 23] that will break the disulfide bonds and allow proteinase K to digest the hair protein and release any trapped nucleic acids. Once released, the DNA can be extracted using the salting-out procedure [25] or organic phenol–chloroform-based extraction [22–24]. Alternative methods include digestion in a buffer containing proteinase K followed by direct PCR [26, 27] or dissolving the hair shaft in sodium hydroxide and, after neutralization, the released DNA is concentrated using filter centrifugation [28].

Because the hair shaft contains very low levels of DNA it is prone to contamination, but unlike many other types of biological evidence with low levels of DNA it is possible to clean the hair shaft prior to DNA extraction. Several methods have been used to clean hair including washing in mild detergents, water and ethanol and also using a mild lysis step in the same way as is used in the differential extraction of semen [29].

Hard tissues

Following murders, terrorist attacks, wars and fatal accidents it is desirable to group together body parts from individuals when fragmentation has occurred and ultimately to identify the deceased. If the time between death and recovery of the body is short then muscle tissues provide a rich source of DNA [30], which can be extracted using, for example, any of the Chelex®, salting-out and organic extraction methods. If, however, the soft tissues are displaying an advanced state of decomposition they will not provide any DNA suitable for analysis. When the cellular structure breaks down during decomposition, enzymes that degrade DNA are released and the DNA within the cell is rapidly digested. This process is accelerated by the action of colonizing bacteria, fungi and insects.

Osteocytes are the most common nucleated cells in the bone matrix (Figure 4.6a). In the teeth, odontoblasts within the dentine and fibroblasts in the cell rich zone of the pulp cavity provide a source of nucleated cells [31] (Figure 4.6b). The hard tissues of the body, bone and teeth provide a refuge for DNA. In addition to the physical barriers, the hydroxyapatite/apatite mineral that is a major component of the hard tissues, stabilizes the DNA which becomes closely bound to the positively charged mineral; this interaction limits the action of degrading enzymes [32].

Hard tissues provide an advantage over other forms of biological material because they have a surface that can be cleaned to remove any contaminating DNA using

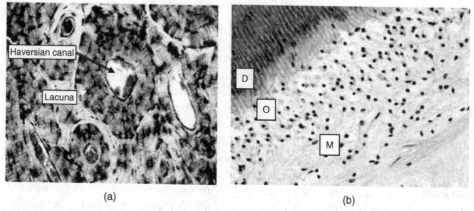

Figure 4.6 Cellular material in bones and teeth. (a) cross-section through a femur: the Haversian canals are surrounded by concentric layers of bone (lamellae); bone cells (osteocytes) occupy lancunae (Image provided by Prof Tim Arnett, Department of Cell & Developmental Biology, University College London, UK). (b) cross-section through a human tooth showing the dentine (D), odontoblast layer (O) and middle part of the dental pulp (M) (Image provided by Dr Marko Vavpotič, Institute of Forensic Medicine, University of Ljubljana, Slovenia)

Figure 4.7 Bone and tooth material can be vigorously cleaned using: (a) abrasion to remove the outer surface and (b) washing in detergent and bleach to remove contaminating materials. (c) Exposure to strong UV light introduces thymine dimers into any contaminating exogenous DNA – preventing amplification during PCR

detergents to remove any soft tissue [33], followed by physical abrasion, soaking in sodium hypochlorite (bleach) [34] (Figure 4.7), trypsin enzyme [35] and exposure to strong ultraviolet light.

After cleaning, the bone/tooth material is normally broken down into a powder by drilling [36] or grinding under liquid nitrogen [37]. The resulting material is then decalcified using 0.5 M EDTA, either before or at the same time as cell lysis [38]. The organic phenol–chloroform and the silica binding extraction methods are commonly used to extract the DNA [7, 37–45]. The process of extracting DNA from bone samples takes longer than with any other type of sample.

Quantification of DNA

After extracting DNA an accurate measurement of the amount of DNA and also the quality of the DNA extract is desirable. Adding the optimum amount of DNA to a PCR will produce the best-quality results in the shortest time; adding too much or not enough DNA will result in a profile that is difficult or even impossible to interpret. This is especially important when profiling forensic samples, when it is very difficult to know the state of preservation of the biological material and also, in many cases, it is difficult to estimate how much cellular material has been collected. It is less important to quantify DNA when using some reference samples – where similar amounts of DNA can be expected to be extracted each time as there are not very many variables. Even so, many laboratories will still quantify the DNA from reference samples as part of their standard analysis. In response to the importance of quantification of samples recovered from the scene of crime, the DNA Advisory Board in the USA adopted rules that made quantification of human DNA mandatory [46].

The quantity of DNA that can be extracted from a sample depends very much on the type of material. Each nucleated cell contains approximately 6 pg of DNA: liquid blood contains 5000−10 000 nucleated blood cells per millilitre; semen contains on average 66 million spermatozoa per millilitre (the average ejaculation produces 2.75 ml of semen) [47]. Biological samples recovered from the scene of crime are not usually in pristine condition and can often consist of a very small number of shed epithelial cells; consequently, the amount of DNA that can be recovered can be extremely low and difficult to quantify.

Visualization on agarose gels

A relatively quick and easy method for assessing both the quantity and the quality of extracted DNA is to visualize it on an agarose gel. Agarose is a polymer that can be poured into a variety of gel forms – mini-gels approximately 10 cm long are sufficient to visualize DNA. The gel is submerged in electrophoresis buffer and the DNA solution is loaded into wells that are formed in the gel by a comb; an electric current is applied across the gel and the negatively charged DNA migrates towards the anode. The agarose gel forms a porous matrix and smaller DNA molecules move through the gel more quickly than do larger DNA molecules. Dyes that intercalate with the DNA double helix, such as ethidium bromide [12], can be added to the gel either before or after electrophoresis, the amount of intercalated dye is proportional to the quantity of DNA. An alternative dye, 4′,6-diamidino-2-phenylindole (DAPI), can be added directly to the DNA before electrophoresis. This migrates through the gel bound to the minor groove of double-stranded DNA [48]. DNA is visualized by placing the gel on a transilluminator that emits UV light at 260 nm. Quantification standards can be run alongside the unknown samples to allow the DNA concentrations to be estimated. In addition to showing the presence of DNA, the size of the extracted DNA molecules can also be estimated. High molecular weight DNA can be seen as a single band while degraded DNA or DNA that has been sheared during extraction appears as a smear. This makes comparison to the standards difficult as the DNA is spread out over a range a random sizes.

The advantages of agarose gel electrophoresis are that it is quick and easy to carry out and also gives an indication of the size of the DNA molecules that have been extracted. The disadvantages are that quantifications are subjective, based on relative band intensities; it is difficult to gauge the amounts of degraded DNA as there is no suitable reference standard; total DNA is detected that can be a mixture of human and microbial DNA, and this can lead to overestimates of the DNA concentration; the sensitivity of the dye under UV light is poor, so low level DNA will not be visible; it cannot be used to quantify samples extracted using the Chelex® method, as this produces single-stranded DNA and the fluorescent dyes that intercalate with the double-stranded DNA do not bind to the single-stranded DNA.

Ultraviolet spectrophotometry

DNA absorbs light maximally at 260 nm. This feature can be used to estimate the amount of DNA in an extract and by measuring a range of wavelengths from 220 nm to 300 nm it is also possible to assess the amount of carbohydrate (maximum absorbance 230 nm) and protein (maximum absorbance 280 nm) that may have co-extracted with the sample. The DNA is placed in a quartz cuvette and light is shone through and the absorbance is measured against a standard. A clean DNA extract will produce a curve as shown in Figure 4.8; if the DNA extract is clean, the ratio of the absorbance at 260 nm and 280 nm should be between 1.8 and 2.0 [12].

Spectrophotometry is commonly used for quantification in molecular biology laboratories but has not been widely adopted by the forensic community. The major disadvantage is that it is difficult to quantify small amounts of DNA accurately using spectrophotometry; also, it is not human specific and other chemicals, for

Figure 4.8 UV absorbance by a solution containing DNA is maximal at 260 nm. The 260:280 ratio of 1.91 indicates that the extract is not contaminated with proteins

example dyes from clothing and humic acids from bone samples, can interfere with the analysis.

Fluorescence spectrophotometry

Ethidium bromide or DAPI can be used to visualize DNA in agarose gels; these are both examples of chemicals that fluoresce at much higher levels when they intercalate with DNA. In addition to staining agarose gels, fluorescent dyes can also be used as an alternative to UV spectrophotometry for DNA quantitation. A range of dyes has been developed that can be used with fluorescent microplate readers and these are very sensitive. The PicoGreen® dye is specific for double-stranded DNA and can detect as little as 25 pg/ml of DNA [46]. When PicoGreen® binds to DNA the fluorescence of the dye increases over 1000-fold; ethidium bromide in comparison increases in fluorescence 50–100-fold when it intercalates with double-stranded DNA [46]. PicoGreen® is very sensitive and is a powerful technique for quantifying total DNA; it does however have the drawback that it is not human specific.

Hybridization

Hybridization-based quantification methods have been widely used in forensic genetics since the early 1990s, in particular a commercially available kit Quantiblot® (Applied Biosystems). Extracted DNA is applied to a positively charged nylon membrane using a slot or dot blot process; the membrane is the exposed to a probe, that is specific to human DNA. A commonly used target was the D17S1 alpha-satellite repeat that is on human chromosome 17 in 500–1000 copies. The probe can be labelled in a number of ways including colorimetric and chemiluminescent.

A series of standards is applied to the membrane, and comparison of the signal from the extracted DNA with the standards allows quantification. The advantage of hybridization-based methods is that the quantification is human specific; agarose gel electrophoresis and spectrophotometry detect total DNA and forensic samples that have been exposed to the environment for any length of time are prone to colonization by bacteria and fungi.

The hybridization systems do suffer from a lack of sensitivity. For samples producing a negative result, in many cases it is still possible to generate a profile after PCR. The analysis of the results is also subjective, leading different operators to come to different conclusions. In addition to the limited sensitivity, the process is labour intensive, taking approximately 2 hours to produce the blot. Hybridization-based methods have been largely replaced by real-time PCR systems.

Real-time PCR

When generating a DNA profile, the PCR products are normally analysed at the end point after 28–34 cycles. It is, however, possible to monitor the generation

Figure 4.9 (a) The TaqMan® quantification system consists of two PCR primers and an internal probe that hybridizes within the amplified region; (b) as the primer extends it encounters the probe, the 5′ exonuclease activity of the *Taq* polymerase degrades the probe: the reporter molecule is no longer in proximity to the quencher and fluoresces

of PCR products as they are generated – real time. This was first developed using ethidium bromide: as PCR products are generated in each cycle, more ethidium bromide intercalates with the double-stranded DNA molecule and fluoresces under UV light. The increase in fluorescence can be detected using a suitable 'camera' [49]. Increasingly sensitive assays have been developed, such as SYBR® Green and the TaqMan® system. Using SYBR® Green, as PCR products are generated, the dye binds to the double-stranded product and the fluorescence increases. The TaqMan® system uses a different approach, with two primers and a probe; the probe is within the region defined by the primers and is labelled on the 5′ end with a fluorescent molecule and on the 3′ end with a molecule that quenches the fluorescence. As the primers are extended by the *Taq* polymerase, one of them meets the probe, which is degraded by the polymerase, releasing the probe and the quencher into solution – efficient quenching of the fluorescent molecules only occurs when they are in close proximity on the probe molecule (Figure 4.9).

As more PCR products are generated, more fluorescent molecules are released and the fluorescence from the sample increases (Figure 4.10). Real-time assays are highly sensitive, human specific and are not labour intensive. In addition to detecting the quantity of DNA they have also been designed to detect PCR inhibition, DNA degradation, male-specific DNA (Y chromosome) and mitochondrial DNA [50–61].

DNA IQ system

A novel approach to quantification is used in the commercially available DNA IQ Isolation System (Promega Corporation). The isolation method is based on salting-out and binding to silica: a very specific amount of silica-coated beads is added to the extraction and these bind a maximum amount of DNA; therefore, when the DNA is eluted from the beads the maximum concentration is known. It has the advantage of combining the extraction and quantification steps and can be semi-automated, but has the disadvantage of not being human specific.

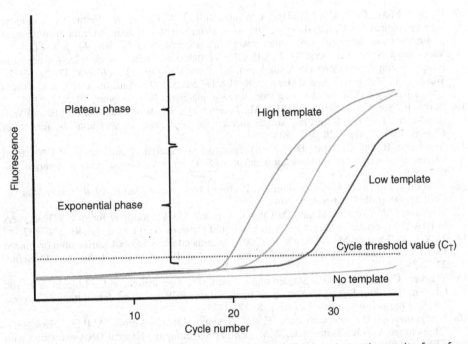

Figure 4.10 Real-time PCR quantification. The schematic diagram shows the results from four different template concentrations: high (——), medium (——), low (——) and no template (——). As the PCR cycles the amount of fluorescence generated increases and each sample that contains template will enter an exponential phase; as the reagents become exhausted each reaction will enter a plateau phase. The cycle threshold value (C_T) is set to detect the point at which the reaction has entered the exponential phase; the cycle number that this occurs will depend on the amount of template DNA added. To determine the concentration of a DNA extract the C_T value is compared to the C_T values from a range of standards

References

1. Aljanabi, S.M. and Martinez, I. (1997) Universal and rapid salt-extraction of high quality genomic DNA for PCR-based techniques. *Nucleic Acids Research*, **25**, 4692–4693.
2. Castella, V., Dimo-Simonin, N., Brandt-Casadevall, C. and Mangin, P. (2006) Forensic evaluation of the QIAshredder/QIAamp DNA extraction procedure. *Forensic Science International*, **156**, 70–73.
3. Greenspoon, S.A., Ban, J.D., Sykes, K., Ballard, E.J., Edler, S.S., Baisden, M. *et al.* (2004) Application of the BioMek (R) 2000 laboratory automation workstation and the DNA IQ (TM) system to the extraction of forensic casework samples. *Journal of Forensic Sciences*, **49**, 29–39.
4. Montpetit, S.A., Fitch, I.T. and O'Donnell, P.T. (2005) A simple automated instrument for DNA extraction in forensic casework. *Journal of Forensic Sciences*, **50**, 555–563.
5. Moss, D., Harbison, S.A. and Saul, D.J. (2003) An easily automated, closed-tube forensic DNA extraction procedure using a thermostable proteinase. *International Journal of Legal Medicine*, **117**, 340–349.
6. Greenspoon, S.A., Scarpetta, M.A., Drayton, M.L. and Turek, S.A. (1998) QIAamp spin columns as a method of DNA isolation for forensic casework. *Journal of Forensic Sciences*, **43**, 1024–1030.

7. Holland, M.M., Cave, C.A., Holland, C.A. and Bille, T.W. (2003) Development of a quality, high throughput DNA analysis procedure for skeletal samples to assist with the identification of victims from the world trade center attacks. *Croatian Medical Journal*, **44**, 264–272.

8. Vandenberg, N. and van Oorschot, R.A.H. (2002) Extraction of human nuclear DNA from feces samples using the QlAamp DNA stool mini kit. *Journal of Forensic Sciences*, **47**, 993–995.

9. Walsh, P.S., Metzger, D.A. and Higuchi, R. (1991) Chelex-100 as a medium for simple extraction of DNA for PCR-based typing from forensic material. *Biotechniques*, **10**, 506–513.

10. Boom, R., Sol, C.J.A., Salimans, M.M.M., Jansen, C.L., Wertheimvandillen, P.M.E. and Vandernoordaa, J. (1990) Rapid and simple method for purification of nucleic-acids. *Journal of Clinical Microbiology*, **28**, 495–503.

11. Vogelstein, B. and Gillespie, D. (1979) Preparative and analytical purification of DNA from agarose. *Proceedings of the National Academy of Sciences of the United States of America*, **76**, 615–619.

12. Sambrook, J., Fritsch, E.F. and Maniatis, T. (1989) *Molecular Cloning: A Laboratory Manual*, Cold Spring Harbor Laboratory Press.

13. Salvador, J.M., Corazon, M. and De Ungria, A. (2004) DNA stability of forensic STR markers in FTA (TM)-extracted buccal DNA of betel-quid chewers. *Oral Oncology*, **40**, 231–232.

14. Tack, L.C., Thomas, M. and Reich, K. (2007) Automated forensic DNA purification optimized for FTA card punches and identifiler STR-based PCR analysis. *Clinics in Laboratory Medicine*, **27**, 183–191.

15. Thacker, C., Phillips, C.P., Syndercombe Court, D., Sensabaugh, G.F., Lincoln, P.J. and Olaisen, B. (2000) Use of FTA cards in small volume PCR reactions. *International Congress Series: Progress in Forensic Genetics*, **8**, 473–475.

16. Wolfgramm, E.D., de Carvalho, F.M., Aguiar, V.R.D., Sartori, M.P.D., Hirschfeld-Campolongo, G.C.R., Tsutsumida, W.M. *et al.* (2009) Simplified buccal DNA extraction with FTA (R) Elute Cards. *Forensic Science International: Genetics*, **3**, 125–127.

17. Natarajan, P., Trinh, T., Mertz, L., Goldsborough, M. and Fox, D.K. (2000) Paper-based archiving of mammalian and plant samples for RNA analysis. *Biotechniques*, **29**, 1328–1333.

18. Brevnov, M.G., Pawar, H.S., Mundt, J., Calandro, L.M., Furtado, M.R. and Shewale, J.G. (2009) Developmental validation of the PrepFiler (TM) Forensic DNA extraction kit for extraction of genomic DNA from biological samples. *Journal of Forensic Sciences*, **54**, 599–607.

19. Holder, F., Eisenberg, A. and Smith, M. (2002) Novel sample collection and purification technology for STR analysis. 16th Meeting of the International Association of Forensic Sciences, pp. 221–224.

20. Gill, P., Jeffreys, A.J. and Werrett, D.J. (1985) Forensic application of DNA fingerprints. *Nature*, **318**, 577–579.

21. Wiegand, P., Schurenkamp, M. and Schutte, U. (1992) DNA extraction from mixtures of body-fluid using mild preferential lysis. *International Journal of Legal Medicine*, **104**, 359–360.

22. Higuchi, R., Vonberoldingen, C.H., Sensabaugh, G.F. and Erlich, H.A. (1988) DNA typing from single hairs. *Nature*, **332**, 543–546.

23. Hellmann, A., Rohleder, U., Schmitter, H. and Wittig, M. (2001) STR typing of human telogen hairs – a new approach. *International Journal of Legal Medicine*, **114**, 269–273.

24. Wilson, M.R., Polanskey, D., Butler, J., Dizinno, J.A., Replogle, J. and Budowle, B. (1995) Extraction, PCR amplification and sequencing of mitochondrial-DNA from human hair shafts. *Biotechniques*, **18**, 662–669.

25. Baker, L.E., McCormick, W.F. and Matteson, K.J. (2001) A silica-based mitochondrial DNA extraction method applied to forensic hair shafts and teeth. *Journal of Forensic Sciences*, **46**, 126–130.

26. Allen, M., Engstrom, A.S., Meyers, S., Handt, O., Saldeen, T. and von Haeseler, A. (1998) Mitochondrial DNA sequencing of shed hairs and saliva on robbery caps: sensitivity and matching probabilities. *Journal of Forensic Sciences*, **43**, 453–464.

27. Vigilant, L. (1999) An evaluation of techniques for the extraction and amplification of DNA from naturally shed hairs. *Biological Chemistry*, **380**, 1329–1331.

28. Graffy, E.A. and Foran, D.R. (2005) A simplified method for mitochondrial DNA extraction from head hair shafts. *Journal of Forensic Sciences*, **50**, 1119–1122.

29. Jehaes, E., Gilissen, A., Cassiman, J.J. and Decorte, R. (1998) Evaluation of a decontamination protocol for hair shafts before mtDNA sequencing. *Forensic Science International*, **94**, 65–71.

30. Bar, W., Kratzer, A., Machler, M. and Schmid, W. (1988) Postmortem stability of DNA. *Forensic Science International*, **39**, 59–70.

31. Gaytmenn, R. and Sweet, D. (2003) Quantification of forensic DNA from various regions of human teeth. *Journal of Forensic Sciences*, **48**, 622–625.

32. Lindahl, T. (1993) Instability and decay of the primary structure of DNA. *Nature*, **362**, 709–715.

33. Arismendi, J.L., Baker, L.E. and Matteson, K.J. (2004) Effects of processing techniques on the forensic DNA analysis of human skeletal remains. *Journal of Forensic Sciences*, **49**, 930–934.

34. Kemp, B.M. and Smith, D.G. (2005) Use of bleach to eliminate contaminating DNA from the surface of bones and teeth. *Forensic Science International*, **154**, 53–61.

35. Li, R., Chapman, S., Thompson, M. and Schwartz, M. (2009) Developing a simple method to process bone samples prior to DNA isolation. *Legal Medicine*, **11**, 76–79.

36. Ginther, C., Isseltarver, L. and King, M.C. (1992) Identifying individuals by sequencing mitochondrial-DNA from teeth. *Nature Genetics*, **2**, 135–138.

37. Loreille, O.M., Dìegoli, T.M., Irwin, J.A., Coble, M.D. and Parsons, T.J. (2007) High efficiency DNA extraction from bone by total demineralization. *Forensic Science International: Genetics*, **1**, 191–195.

38. Fisher, D.L., Holland, M.M., Mitchell, L., Sledzik, P.S., Wilcox, A.W., Wadhams, M. *et al.* (1993) Extraction, evaluation, and amplification of DNA from decalcified and undecalcified United-States civil-war bone. *Journal of Forensic Sciences*, **38**, 60–68.

39. Bille, T., Wingrove, R., Holland, M., Holland, C., Cave, C. and Schumm, J. (2004) Novel method of DNA extraction from bones assisted DNA identification of World Trade Center victims, in *Progress in Forensic Genetics*, vol. **10**, Elsevier, pp. 553–555.

40. Crainic, K., Paraire, F., Leterreux, M., Durigon, M., de Mazancourt and P. (2002) Skeletal remains presumed submerged in water for three years identified using PCR-STR analysis. *Journal of Forensic Sciences*, **47**, 1025–1027.

41. Goodwin, W., Linacre, A. and Vanezis, P. (1999) The use of mitochondrial DNA and short tandem repeat typing in the identification of air crash victims. *Electrophoresis*, **20**, 1707–1711.

42. Goodwin, W., McFarlane, J. and Roberts, J. (2003) The identification of a US serviceman recovered from the Holy Loch, Scotland. *Science and Justice*, **43**, 45–47.

43. Holland, M.M., Fisher, D.L., Mitchell, L.G., Rodriguez, W.C., Canik, J.J., Merril, C.R. *et al.* (1993) Mitochondrial-DNA sequence-analysis of human skeletal remains – identification of remains from the Vietnam-War. *Journal of Forensic Sciences*, **38**, 542–553.

44. Davoren, J., Vanek, D., Konjhodzic, R., Crews, J., Huffine, E. and Parsons, T.J. (2007) Highly effective DNA extraction method for nuclear short tandem repeat testing of skeletal remains from mass graves. *Croatian Medical Journal*, **48**, 478–485.

45. Edson, S.M., Ross, J.P., Coble, M.D., Parsons, T.J. and Barritt, S.M. (2004) Naming the dead-confronting the realities of rapid identification of degraded skeletal remains. *Forensic Science Review*, **16**, 63–90.

46. Nicklas, J.A. and Buel, E. (2003) Quantification of DNA in forensic samples. *Analytical and Bioanalytical Chemistry*, **376**, 1160–1167.

47. Carlsen, E., Giwercman, A., Keiding, N. and Skakkebaek, N.E. (1992) Evidence for decreasing quality of semen during past 50 years. *British Medical Journal*, **305**, 609–613.

48. Buel, E. (1995) The Use of DAPI as a replacement for ethidium-bromide in forensic DNA analysis. *Journal of Forensic Sciences*, **40**, 275–278.

49. Higuchi, R., Fockler, C., Dollinger, G. and Watson, R. (1993) Kinetic PCR analysis – real-time monitoring of DNA amplification reactions. *Bio-Technology*, **11**, 1026–1030.

50. Barbisin, M., Fang, R., O'Shea, C.E., Calandro, L.M., Furtado, M.R. and Shewale, J.G. (2009) Developmental validation of the quantifiler((R)) duo DNA quantification kit for simultaneous quantification of total human and human male DNA and detection of PCR inhibitors in biological samples. *Journal of Forensic Sciences*, **54**, 305–319.

51. Horsman, K.M., Hickey, J.A., Cotton, R.W., Landers, J.P. and Maddox, L.O. (2006) Development of a human-specific real-time PCR assay for the simultaneous quantitation of total genomic and male DNA. *Journal of Forensic Sciences*, **51**, 758–765.
52. Hudlow, W.R., Chong, M.D., Swango, K.L., Timken, M.D. and Buoncristiani, M.R. (2008) A quadruplex real-time qPCR assay for the simultaneous assessment of total human DNA, human male DNA, DNA degradation and the presence of PCR inhibitors in forensic samples: A diagnostic tool for STR typing. *Forensic Science International: Genetics*, **2**, 108–125.
53. Kontanis, E.J. and Reed, F.A. (2006) Evaluation of real-time PCR amplification efficiencies to detect PCR inhibitors. *Journal of Forensic Sciences*, **51**, 795–804.
54. Nicklas, J.A. and Buel, E. (2003) Development of an Alu-based, real-time PCR method for quantitation of human DNA in forensic samples. *Journal of Forensic Sciences*, **48**, 936–944.
55. Nicklas, J.A. and Buel, E. (2006) Simultaneous determination of total human and male DNA using a duplex real-time PCR assay. *Journal of Forensic Sciences*, **51**, 1005–1015.
56. Nielsen, K., Chong, M.D., Swango, K.L., Timken, M.D. and Buoncristiani, M.R. (2008) Comparison of five DNA quantification methods. *Forensic Science International: Genetics*, **2**, 226–230.
57. Swango, K.L., Hudlow, W.R., Timken, M.D. and Buoncristiani, M.R. (2007) Developmental validation of a multiplex qPCR assay for assessing the quantity and quality of nuclear DNA in forensic samples. *Forensic Science International*, **170**, 35–45.
58. Swango, K.L., Timken, M.D., Chong, M.D. and Buoncristiani, M.R. (2006) A quantitative PCR assay for the assessment of DNA degradation in forensic samples. *Forensic Science International*, **158**, 14–26.
59. Walker, J.A., Hedges, D.J., Perodeau, B.P., Landry, K.E., Stoilova, N., Laborde, M.E. *et al.* (2005) Multiplex polymerase chain reaction for simultaneous quantitation of human nuclear, mitochondrial, and male Y-chromosome DNA: application in human identification. *Analytical Biochemistry*, **337**, 89–97.
60. Walker, J.A., Hughes, D.A., Hedges, D.J., Anders, B.A., Laborde, M.E., Shewale, J. *et al.* (2004) Quantitative PCR for DNA identification based on genome-specific interspersed repetitive elements. *Genomics*, **83**, 518–527.
61. Westring, C.G., Kristinsson, R., Gilbert, D.M. and Danielson, P.B. (2007) Validation of reduced-scale reactions for the Quantifiler (TM) human DNA kit. *Journal of Forensic Sciences*, **52**, 1035–1043.

5 Polymerase chain reaction

In 1985 a new method – the polymerase chain reaction (PCR) – was reported [1–3]. PCR can amplify a specific region of DNA by copying the locus exponentially. The method has revolutionized all areas of molecular biology, including forensic genetics, as extremely small quantities of DNA can be analysed. Under optimal conditions, DNA can be amplified from a single cell [4, 5]. The increased sensitivity of DNA profiling using PCR has had a dramatic effect on the types of forensic sample that can be used, and it is now possible to analyse trace evidence and highly degraded samples successfully – albeit with less than 100% success.

The evolution of PCR-based profiling in forensic genetics

PCR technology was rapidly incorporated into forensic analysis. The first PCR-based tool for forensic casework amplified the polymorphic HLA-DQα locus (the α subunit of the DQ protein is part of the major histocompatibility complex) [6]. It was used for the first time in casework in 1988 to analyse the skeletal remains of a 3-year-old girl [7, 8]. The DQα system's major drawback was that it had a limited power of discrimination.

Minisatellites (VNTRs) were widely used in casework but required a relatively large amount of DNA. In an attempt to overcome this limitation, PCR technology was applied to the analysis of VNTR loci, and alleles between 5 kb and 10 kb could be faithfully amplified from fresh biological material [9]. However, it was of limited value for many forensic samples, which often contained small amounts of DNA that was highly degraded. To overcome the problems caused by degradation, tandem repeats, called amplified fragment length polymorphisms (AMP-FLPs) that were smaller than 1 kb were selected for PCR based analysis [10–15]. However, as with VNTRs, their use was limited in forensic contexts because of the size of the larger alleles, which were difficult to analyse in degraded samples. By the early 1990s, a large number of STRs had been characterized [16]. The STR loci were simpler and shorter than VNTRs and AMP-FLPs, and were more suitable for the analysis of biological samples recovered from crime scenes [17]. The STR markers were not individually as discriminating as the VNTR and AMP-FLPs, but had a major advantage that several of them could be analysed together in a multiplex reaction.

An Introduction to Forensic Genetics Second Edition   William Goodwin, Adrian Linacre and Sibte Hadi
© 2011 John Wiley & Sons, Ltd

The STR markers have become the genetic polymorphism of choice in forensic genetics and PCR is a vital part of the analytical process.

DNA replication: the basis of the PCR

PCR takes advantage of the enzymatic processes of DNA replication. During every cell cycle the entire DNA content of a cell is duplicated. This copying of DNA can be replicated outside the cell, *in vitro*, to amplify specific regions of DNA.

The components of PCR

PCR has the following components: template DNA, at least two primers, a thermostable DNA polymerase such as *Taq* polymerase, magnesium chloride, deoxynucleotide triphosphates and a buffer.

Template DNA

The amount of DNA added to a PCR depends on the sensitivity of the reaction: for most forensic purposes the PCR is highly optimized so that it will work with low levels of template. Most commercial kits require between 0.5 ng and 2.5 ng of extracted DNA for optimum results. This represents between 166 and 833 copies of the haploid human genome; one copy of the human genome contains approximately 3 pg of DNA. Most forensic profiling can be carried out successfully with fewer templates – even below 100 pg or 33 copies of the genome [18, 19]; however, the interpretation of profiles can become more complex as the amount of template DNA is reduced.

Taq DNA polymerase

The first PCRs were carried out using a DNA polymerase that was isolated from *Esherichia coli;* in each cycle of the PCR the enzyme was inactivated by the high temperatures in the denaturation phase and fresh enzyme had to be added [1–3]. Fortunately, this is no longer necessary. Scientists were able to isolate the DNA polymerases from the thermophilic bacteria, *Thermus aquaticus* [20], which was discovered in the 1960s in the hot springs of Yellowstone National Park, USA. The *Taq* polymerase enzyme can tolerate the high temperatures that are involved in the PCR and works optimally at 72 °C–80 °C [21]. Using the thermostable enzyme greatly simplifies the PCR procedure and also increases the specificity, sensitivity and yield of the reaction [21]. The *Taq* polymerase enzyme exhibits significant activity at room temperature that can lead to the creation of non-specific PCR products; adding the enzyme to a pre-heated 'hot start' reaction reduces the non-specific binding and again improves the specificity and yield of a PCR [22]. Modifications to the commonly used *Taq* polymerase led to the development of the AmpliTaq Gold®

polymerase (Applied Biosystems). The enzyme is inactive when it is first added to the PCR; it only becomes active after incubation at 95 °C for approximately 10 minutes [23]. This 'hot start' enzyme allows the PCR to start at an elevated temperature and minimizes the non-specific binding that can occur at lower temperatures [24].

Primers

The primers used in PCR define the region of the genome that will be analysed. Primers are short synthetic pieces of DNA that anneal to the template molecule either side of the target region. The primer sequences are therefore limited to some degree by the DNA sequence that flanks the target sequence. Figure 5.1 illustrates the sequence and positioning of two primers that are used to amplify the D16S539 locus in one of the commercially available kits for analysing STR loci (Promega Corporation).

When designing primers for forensic analysis it is important that they will bind to conserved regions of DNA and therefore effectively amplify human DNA from all populations [25], while at the same time not binding to the DNA of other species. When designing a multiplex PCR, the allelic size ranges are also important considerations for the position of the primer binding sites.

There are a number of basic guidelines for primer design. Primers are normally between 18 and 30 nucleotides long, and have a balanced number of G/C and A/T nucleotides. A primer should not be self-complementary or be complementary to any of the other primers that are in the reaction. Self-complementary regions will result in the primer pairing with itself to form a loop, whereas primers that are complementary will bind to each other to form primer dimers.

The temperature at which primers anneal to the template DNA depends upon their length and sequence; most primers are designed to anneal between 50 °C and 65 °C. A basic rule of thumb can be used when designing primers to estimate the melting temperature (the temperature at which half of a particular DNA duplex

```
 01  ggagctgggg ggtctaagag cttgtaaaaa gtgtacaagt gccagatgct cgttgtgcac
 61  aaatctaaat gcagaaaagc actgaaagaa gaatcccgaa aaccacagtt cccattttta
121  tatgggagca aacaaagcag atcccaagct cttcctcttc cctagatcaa tacagacaga
181  cagacaggtg GATAGATAGA TAGATAGATA GATAGATAGA TAGATAGATA GATAtcattg
241  aaagacaaaa cagagatgga tgatagatac atgcttacag atgcacacac aaacgctaaa
```

Forward Primer: 5'- GGG GGT CTA AGA GCT TGT AAA AAG - 3'

Reverse Primer: 5'- GTT TGT GTG TGC ATC TGT AAG CAT - 3'

Figure 5.1 The forward and reverse primers that are used to amplify the short tandem repeat (STR) locus D16S539 in the Promega Powerplex™ 1.2 Kit are shown; the position that they bind to within the sequence is indicated by the arrows. The target sequence is shown in bold: the position of the primers around either side of the target determines the length of the PCR product. The example contains 11 repeats of the core GATA sequence (see Chapter 6 for details of STRs) will become dissociated): for each A or T in the primer 2 °C is added to the melting temperature and for each C or G 4 °C is added; Cs and Gs will bind to the complementary nucleotide with three hydrogen bonds and are therefore more thermodynamically stable. To estimate the annealing temperature 5 °C, is subtracted from the melting temperature. PCR primers can be designed manually or using more sophisticated algorithms with the aid of software such as Oligo [26], Primer3 [27] and OligoCalc [28].

Magnesium chloride, nucleotide triphosphates and reaction buffer

$MgCl_2$ is a critical component of the PCR. The primers bind to the template DNA to form a primer–template duplex: $MgCl_2$ stabilizes the interaction. The concentration of $MgCl_2$ is typically between 1.5 mM and 2.5 mM; the template–primer stability increases with higher concentrations of $MgCl_2$. A balance is required between the concentration of $MgCl_2$ and the annealing temperature. The *Taq* polymerase also requires magnesium to be present in order to function.

The building blocks for the PCR are deoxynucleotide triphosphates, which are incorporated into the nascent DNA strand during replication. The four nucleotides are in the PCR in equal concentration, normally 200 μM. The reaction buffer maintains optimal pH and salt conditions for the reaction.

The PCR process

The PCR amplifies specific regions of template DNA. The power of the technique is illustrated in Table 5.1. In theory, a single molecule can be amplified 1 billion-fold by 30 cycles of amplification; in practice, the PCR is not 100% efficient but does still produce tens of millions of copies of the target sequence [21].

The amplification of DNA occurs in the cycling phase of PCR, which consists of three stages (Figure 5.2): denaturation, annealing and extension. In the denaturation stage the reaction is heated to 94 °C; this causes the double-stranded DNA molecule to 'melt' forming two single-stranded molecules. DNA melts at this temperature because the hydrogen bonds that hold the two strands of the DNA molecule together are relatively weak. As the temperature is lowered, typically to between 50 °C and 65 °C, the oligonucleotide primers anneal to the template. The primers are in molar excess to the template strands and bind to the complementary sequences before the template DNA reassociates to form double-stranded DNA. After the primers have annealed, the temperature is increased to 72 °C, which is in the optimum temperature range for the *Taq* polymerase. Nucleotides are added to the nascent DNA strand at the rate of approximately 40–60 per second [29, 30]. The enzyme catalyses the addition of nucleotides to the 3′ ends of the primers using the original DNA strand as a template; it has a high processivity, catalysing the addition of approximately 50 nucleotides to the nascent DNA strand before the enzyme dissociates; several *Taq* polymerase enzymes will associate and disassociate during the extension phase of longer PCR products.

Table 5.1 The PCR reaction can theoretically multiply DNA over 1 billion-fold after 32 cycles; in reality it is not 100% efficient but is still extremely powerful

Cycle	Number of PCR products
1	0
2	0
3	2
4	4
5	8
6	16
7	32
8	64
9	128
10	256
20	262 144
28[1]	67 108 864
30	268 435 456
32[2]	1 073 741 824
34[3]	4 294 967 296

[1] Standard cycle number using Applied Biosystems SGM Plus and Identifiler Kits.
[2] Standard cycle number using Promega PowerPlex 16 Kit.
[3] Maximum number of cycles normally used in forensic analysis.

Double-stranded DNA template molecule –hydrogen bonds hold the two strands together

The temperature is increased to 95 °C. This causes the hydrogen bonds to break and results in two denatured single-stranded DNA molecules.

Two single-stranded DNA molecules

The temperature is reduced to 50 °C–60 °C allowing primers to anneal to complementary sequences. The two primers must anneal to the two different strands and must be extended towards each other.

Hydrogen bonds stabilize the template–primer interaction. The arrow head indicates the direction of primer extension

The temperature is increased to 72 °C. The enzyme *Taq* polymerase finds the free ends of the primers (indicated by the arrow heads) and starts to incorporate nucleotides that are complementary to the template strand.

The end product is two double-stranded copies of the template DNA

Figure 5.2 The PCR reaction – each PCR cycle consists of three phases: denaturing, annealing and extension

The normal range of cycles for a PCR is between 28 and 32. In extreme cases, where the amount of target DNA is very low the cycle number can be increased to up to 34 cycles. It has been demonstrated that going above this cycle number does not increase the likelihood of obtaining a profile but does increase the probability of artefacts forming during the PCR [18]. Using 34 cycles is known as low copy number (LCN) PCR[1] and it is sparingly employed, as extreme precautions have to be taken to reduce the chance of contamination; the more cycles the higher the chance of detecting contaminating DNA. The interpretation of the profiles generated using a high cycle number also become more complex.

Following the cycling phase the reaction is incubated between 60 °C and 72 °C for up to 1 hour. In addition to the template-dependent synthesis of DNA, the *Taq* polymerase also adds an additional residue to the 3′ end of extended DNA molecule, this is non-template dependent [31]; the incubation at the end of the reaction is to ensure that the non-template addition is complete. The conditions of a typical PCR are shown below in Figure 5.3.

The PCR requires tightly controlled thermal conditions and these are achieved by using a thermocycler. This consists of a conducting metal block that contains heating and cooling elements with wells that accommodate the plastic reaction tubes. The temperature of the PCR block is controlled by a small microprocessor. Most thermocyclers also contain a lid, which is heated to over 100 °C; this prevents the reaction evaporating and condensing on the cooler lid and thereby maintains the reaction volume, thus keeping the concentration of the reaction components stable throughout the PCR.

After amplification the results of a PCR can be visualized on an agarose gel. In a reaction that amplifies only one locus a single band should be detected[2] (Figure 5.4).

PCR inhibition

When analysing forensic samples a problem that can be encountered is inhibition of the PCR [32]. DNA extraction methods do not produce pure DNA; some chemicals

1 Hold	3 Tmp 28 cycles	2 Holds
94.0	94.0	
11:00	1:00	59.0	72.0	60.0
		1:00	1:00	65:00	4.0
				∞

Method: SGM+

Figure 5.3 A typical PCR programme involves three phases: a pre-incubation at 94 °C, which activates the AmpliTaq Gold® polymerase; the cycling phase; and a terminal incubation that maximizes the non-template addition at the end of the amplification. The programme shown is for amplification using the SGM Plus® (see Chapter 6)

---

[1] Note: The term low copy number PCR is now commonly referred to as low template number PCR.

[2] Note: An exception would be when the target locus contains alleles of varying length, such as VNTRs, AMP-FLPs and STRs.

Figure 5.4 (a) The target sequence on the template DNA molecule has been amplified using two different primer pairs: using primers a +c generates a 500 bp product and the a + b primer pair leads to a 200 bp product. (b) Following amplification of template DNA in two separate reactions the products were separated on a 2% agarose gel and stained with ethidium bromide. The amplified products can be seen in lane 2 (200 bp) and lane 3 (500 bp); lane 1 contains a 100 bp ladder

will co-purify and in some cases inhibit the *Taq* polymerase. Potent inhibitors of the *Taq* polymerase include haem compounds from blood [33–38]; bile salts and complex polysaccharides from faeces and plant material [38–41]; humic substances from soil, which is commonly co-extracted from bone [36, 42–44]; urea from urine [38, 45–47]; melanin from hair and skin [48]; blue dye in clothing such as denim, called indigo [49]; collagen from tissue and bones [50]; and high concentrations of ions, in particular calcium and magnesium [46]. EDTA is used in high concentrations for the isolation of DNA from bone and will also inhibit PCR unless removed as it binds ions such as magnesium ions that are essential for PCR [36].

Extraction methods have been developed to remove commonly encountered PCR inhibitors and, for example the silica-based methods that are commonly used in forensic analysis are effective at removing most inhibitors, whereas the methods that produce a cruder extract such as the Chelex® resin are more prone to inhibition. When it is not possible to remove all the potential inhibitors from a DNA extract, the addition of the protein bovine serum albumin (BSA) to the PCR can in many cases prevent or reduce the inhibition of the *Taq* polymerase. The BSA acts as a binding site for some inhibitors and can competitively remove or reduce the concentration of the inhibitor [33, 36].

The action of inhibitors can be detected, for example by spiking a PCR with a known amount of DNA; this alerts the analyst that further purification steps are required [51]. PCR inhibition can also be detected using real-time DNA quantification (see Chapter 4).

Sensitivity and contamination

The great advantage of PCR is that it will amplify DNA from a template of only a few cells. This high level of sensitivity can also be a potential disadvantage, as DNA from incidental sources can be present and contamination can be introduced. Throughout the handling and analysis of DNA samples, extreme care needs to be taken to minimize the chance of introducing this extraneous DNA.

When samples are collected from the scene of an incident, there may be cellular material from persons who had been present at the scene prior to the incident and hence DNA profiles will be generated from people unconnected with the incident. This type of DNA can be termed as incidental as it is not a contamination of the samples. At the time of the incident there is an opportunity for transfer from the perpetrator, and it is this cellular material that is pertinent to the investigation. Consider an event such as theft from a house. Prior to the incident there will be cellular material from the owners and from any recent visitors. At the time of the break in there may be transfer from the burglar. If the incident is discovered by a neighbour, then they will introduce their cellular material after the incident and prior to the scene being secured. When the police are called they have the potential to introduce their cellular material. Once the scene is secured then those entering should be wearing full protection to minimize the opportunity for transfer of their cellular material [52, 53]. If there is any introduction of DNA from those at the crime scene, during collection and transportation, or from laboratory staff, then this is considered as contamination.

The PCR laboratory

Once evidential samples have reached the forensic laboratory there is further potential to introduce contamination. A fundamental feature of PCR laboratories, to reduce the possibility of introducing contamination, is that they are clearly divided into pre- and post-PCR areas (Figure 5.5).

Pre-PCR

Once the samples reach the laboratory, potential contamination comes from the reagents, equipment and the forensic scientists undertaking the analysis. To prevent contamination being introduced from the scientist, protective clothing is worn,

Figure 5.5 The PCR laboratory is designed so that the work flows through the different processes in one direction starting with sample reception and forensic biology and finishing with the post-PCR analysis. The samples are passed through air-lock hatches to minimize the possibility of any material being transferred from post-PCR to pre-PCR areas. Access to the pre- and post-PCR laboratories is through different changing areas and dedicated staff will work in either pre- or post-PCR areas. Positive air pressure in pre-PCR areas and negative pressure in post-PCR rooms also reduces the possibility of introducing any contamination into the pre-PCR areas

including a lab coat, gloves, a face mask, safety glasses/visor and a head cover. Even with these precautions it is still possible to get the scientist's DNA profile showing up; a database of all the people who enter/work in the laboratory can be used to detect when contamination could have been introduced within the laboratory.[3]

When laboratories are engaged in analysing both samples from suspects and from crime scenes, it is important to have dedicated areas for the two classes of sample; this prevents any potential cross-contamination of the crime scene and suspect DNA. Special dedicated facilities may also be used when dealing with samples that contain very small amounts of DNA, such as hair shafts.

DNA extraction and PCR set-up are commonly carried out in specialized clean hoods that provide a very controlled environment. The hoods have stainless steel surfaces and are easy to keep clean; they have filtered air to prevent any dust or other contaminant getting into the reaction. The pipetting of any liquids involved in the extraction and PCR set-up is performed using pipette tips with barriers to prevent any DNA carry-over contamination.

---

[3] Note: Databases may also contain the DNA profiles of Police Officers and Crime Scene Investigators who could potentially contaminate crime scenes with their own DNA.

During the DNA extraction process negative control extractions must always be carried out to monitor for contamination; positive controls that involve extracting material similar to the casework samples, for example buccal swabs or bloodstains, can be carried out to monitor that the extraction and amplification procedures are working efficiently. The PCR set-up introduces another positive and negative control: the positive control involves setting up a PCR with DNA of known origin and whose profile is known. Successful analysis demonstrates that the PCR worked. In the negative control PCR, water replaces the DNA to monitor for contamination in the reagents or introduced during the PCR set-up.

Post-PCR

The most potent source of contamination is previously amplified PCR products. Following a PCR there are millions of copies of the target sequence that can potentially contaminate subsequent reactions. Each time a PCR tube is opened there is some aerosol spray, and a single droplet of aerosol will contain thousands of copies of the amplified target, resulting in transfer of some of the amplified product. The fundamental feature of any laboratory that engages in PCR analysis is that there must be physical separation of the pre-PCR and the post-PCR analysis to minimize the possibility of contaminating DNA extractions and PCR set-ups with amplified material. In addition to the two physical spaces, there should also be dedicated equipment, protective clothing and reagents for each area. There must be a unidirectional work flow through the laboratory; PCR products must never be brought back into the pre-PCR part of the laboratory. There must also be temporal separation of tasks; it is not possible for a scientist who has been working in the post-PCR to then work in the pre-PCR area without the possibility of introducing contamination; an overnight break before returning to the pre-PCR area is normally recommended. Larger laboratories will have scientists who are dedicated to only the pre- or the post-PCR analysis.

Further reading

Dieffenbach, C.W. and Dveksler, G.S. (2003) *PCR Primer: A Laboratory Manual*, 2nd edn, Cold Spring Harbor Laboratory Press.

WWW resources

Primer3 – PCR primer design software: http://primer3.sourceforge.net/
OligoCalc – oligonucleotide properties calculator: http://www.basic.northwestern.edu/biotools/oligocalc.html

References

1. Mullis, K., Faloona, F., Scharf, S., Saiki, R., Horn, G. and Erlich, H. (1986) Specific enzymatic amplification of DNA in vitro – the polymerase chain-reaction. *Cold Spring Harbor Symposia on Quantitative Biology*, **51**, 263–273.

2. Mullis, K.B. and Faloona, F.A. (1987) Specific synthesis of DNA in vitro via a polymerase-catalyzed chain-reaction. *Methods in Enzymology*, **155**, 335–350.
3. Saiki, R.K., Scharf, S., Faloona, F., Mullis, K.B., Horn, G.T. and Erlich, H.A. *et al.* (1985) Enzymatic amplification of beta-globin genomic sequences and restriction site analysis for diagnosis of sickle-cell anemia. *Science*, **230**, 1350–1354.
4. Li, H.H., Cui, X.F. and Arnheim, N. (1990) Direct electrophoretic detection of the allelic state of single DNA-molecules in human sperm by using the polymerase chain-reaction. *Proceedings of the National Academy of Sciences of the United States of America*, **87**, 4580–4584.
5. Li, H.H., Gyllensten, U.B., Cui, X.F., Saiki, R.K., Erlich, H.A. and Arnheim, N. (1988) Amplification and analysis of DNA-sequences in single human-sperm and diploid-cells. *Nature*, **335**, 414–417.
6. Saiki, R.K., Bugawan, T.L., Horn, G.T., Mullis, K.B. and Erlich, H.A. (1986) Analysis of enzymatically amplified beta-globin and HLA-DQ-alpha DNA with allele-specific oligonucleotide probes. *Nature*, **324**, 163–166.
7. Blake, E., Crim, D., Mihalovich, J., Higuchi, R., Walsh, P.S. and Erlich, H. (1992) Polymerase chain-reaction (PCR) amplification and human-leukocyte antigen (HLA)-DQ-alpha oligonucleotide typing on biological evidence samples – casework experience. *Journal of Forensic Science*, **37**, 700–726.
8. Stoneking, M., Hedgecock, D., Higuchi, R.G., Vigilant, L. and Erlich, H.A. (1991) Population variation of human mtDNA control region sequences detected by enzymatic amplification and sequence-specific oligonucleotide probes. *American Journal of Human Genetics*, **48**, 370–382.
9. Jeffreys, A.J., Wilson, V., Neumann, R. and Keyte, J. (1988) Amplification of human minisatellites by the polymerase chain-reaction – towards DNA fingerprinting of single cells. *Nucleic Acids Research*, **16**, 10953–10971.
10. Boerwinkle, E., Xiong, W.J., Fourest, E. and Chan, L. (1989) Rapid typing of tandemly repeated hypervariable loci by the polymerase chain-reaction – application to the apolipoprotein-B 3' hypervariable region. *Proceedings of the National Academy of Sciences of the United States of America*, **86**, 212–216.
11. Budowle, B., Chakraborty, R., Giusti, A.M., Eisenberg, A.J. and Allen, R.C. (1991) Analysis of the VNTR locus D1S80 by the PCR followed by high-resolution page. *American Journal of Human Genetics*, **48**, 137–144.
12. Horn, G.T., Richards, B. and Klinger, K.W. (1989) Amplification of a highly polymorphic VNTR segment by the polymerase chain-reaction. *Nucleic Acids Research*, **17**, 2140–2140.
13. Kasai, K., Nakamura, Y. and White, R. (1990) Amplification of a variable number of tandem repeats (VNTR) locus (PMCT118) by the polymerase chain-reaction (PCR) and its application to forensic-science. *Journal of Forensic Science*, **35**, 1196–1200.
14. Rand, S. Puers, C., Skowasch, K., Wiegand, P., Budowle, B. and Brinkmann, B. (1992) Population-genetics and forensic efficiency data of 4 AMP-FLPs. *International Journal of Legal Medicine*, **104**, 329–333.
15. Sajantila, A., Strom, M., Budowle, B., Karhunen, P.J. and Peltonen, L. (1991) The polymerase chain-reaction and postmortem forensic identity testing – application of amplified D1S80 and HLA-DQ-alpha loci to the identification of fire victims. *Forensic Science International*, **51**, 23–34.
16. Edwards, A., Civitello, A., Hammond, H.A. and Caskey, C.T. (1991) DNA typing and genetic-mapping with trimeric and tetrameric tandem repeats. *American Journal of Human Genetics*, **49**, 746–756.
17. Hagelberg, E., Gray, I.C. and Jeffreys, A.J. (1991) Identification of the skeletal remains of a murder victim by DNA analysis. *Nature*, **352**, 427–429.
18. Gill, P. (2001) Application of low copy number DNA profiling. *Croatian Medical Journal*, **42**, 229–232.
19. Gill, P., Whitaker, J., Flaxman, C., Brown, N. and Buckleton, J. (2000) An investigation of the rigor of interpretation rules for STRs derived from less than 100 pg of DNA. *Forensic Science International*, **112**, 17–40.
20. Chien, A., Edgar, D.B. and Trela, J.M. (1976) Deoxyribonucleic-acid polymerase from extreme thermophile thermus-aquaticus. *Journal of Bacteriology*, **127**, 1550–1557.

21. Saiki, R.K., Gelfand, D.H., Stoffel, S., Scharf, S.J., Higuchi, R., Horn, GT. *et al.* (1988) Primer-directed enzymatic amplification of DNA with a thermostable DNA-polymerase. *Science*, **239**, 487–491.

22. Daquila, R.T., Bechtel, L.J., Videler, J.A., Eron, J.J., Gorczyca, P. and Kaplan, J.C. (1991) Maximizing sensitivity and specificity of PCR by preamplification heating. *Nucleic Acids Research*, **19**, 3749–3749.

23. Birch, D.E., Kolmodin, L., Laird, W.J., McKinney, N., Wong, J., Young, K.K.Y. *et al.* (1996) Simplified hot start PCR. *Nature*, **381**, 445–446.

24. Moretti, T., Koons, B., Budowle, B. (1998) Enhancement of PCR amplification yield and specificity using AmpliTaq Gold (TM) DNA polymerase. *Biotechniques*, **25**, 716–722.

25. Budowle, B., Masibay, A., Anderson, S.J., Barna, C., Biega, L., Brenneke, S. *et al.* (2001) STR primer concordance study. *Forensic Science International*, **124**, 47–54.

26. Rychlik, W. and Rhoads, R.E. (1989) A computer-program for choosing optimal oligonu-cleotides for filter hybridization, sequencing and in vitro amplification of DNA. *Nucleic Acids Research*, **17**, 8543–8551.

27. Rozen, S. and Skaletsky, H.J. (2000) Primer3 on the WWW for general users and for biologist programmers, in *Bioinformatics Methods and Protocols: Methods in Molecular Biology* (eds S. Krawetz and S. Misener), Humana Press, pp. 365–386.

28. Kibbe, W.A. (2007) OligoCalc: an online oligonucleotide properties calculator. *Nucleic Acids Research*, **35**, W43–W46.

29. Applied Biosystems. Feature Guide for PCR Enzymes. http://www3.appliedbiosystems.com/cms/groups/mcb_marketing/documents/generaldocuments/cms_042363.pdf (accessed July 2010).

30. Takagi, M., Nishioka, M., Kakihara, H., Kitabayashi, M., Inoue, H., Kawakami, B. *et al.* (1997) Characterization of DNA polymerase from Pyrococcus sp. strain KOD1 and its application to PCR. *Applied and Environmental Microbiology*, **63**, 4504–4510.

31. Clark, J.M. (1988) Novel non-templated nucleotide addition-reactions catalyzed by prokaryotic and eukaryotic DNA-polymerases. *Nucleic Acids Research*, **16**, 9677–9686.

32. Wilson, I.G. (1997) Inhibition and facilitation of nucleic acid amplification. *Applied and Environmental Microbiology*, **63**, 3741–3751.

33. Akane, A., Matsubara, K., Nakamura, H., Takahashi, S. and Kimura, K. (1994) Identification of the heme compound copurified with deoxyribonucleic-acid (DNA) from bloodstains, a major Inhibitor of polymerase chain-reaction (PCR) amplification. *Journal of Forensic Science*, **39**, 362–372.

34. Akane, A., Matsubara, K., Nakamura, H., Takahashi, S., Kimura, K. (1993) Purification of forensic specimens for the polymerase chain-reaction (PCR) analysis. *Journal of Forensic Science*, **38**, 691–701.

35. Defranchis, R., Cross, N.C.P., Foulkes, N.S. and Cox, T.M. (1988) A potent inhibitor of taq polymerase copurifies with human genomic DNA. *Nucleic Acids Research*, **16**, 10355–10355.

36. Kreader, C.A. (1996) Relief of amplification inhibition in PCR with bovine serum albumin or T4 gene 32 protein. *Applied and Environmental Microbiology*, **62**, 1102–1106.

37. Comey, C.T., Koons, B.W., Presley, K.W., Smerick, J.B., Sobieralski, C.A., Stanley, D.M. (1994) DNA extraction strategies for amplified fragment length polymorphism analysis. *Journal of Forensic Science*, **39**, 1254–1269.

38. Radstrom, P., Knutsson, R., Wolffs, P., Lovenklev, M. and Lofstrom, C. (2004) Pre-PCR processing – strategies to generate PCR-compatible samples. *Molecular Biotechnology*, **26**, 133–146.

39. Lantz, P.G., Matsson, M., Wadstrom, T. and Radstrom, P. (1997) Removal of PCR inhibitors from human faecal samples through the use of an aqueous two-phase system for sample preparation prior to PCR. *Journal of Microbiological Methods*, **28**, 159–167.

40. Monteiro, L., Bonnemaison, D., Vekris, A., Petry, K.G., Bonnet, J., Vidal, R. *et al.* (1997) Complex polysaccharides as PCR inhibitors in feces: Helicobacter pylori model. *Journal of Clinical Microbiology*, **35**, 995–998.

41. Rouhibakhsh, A., Priya, J., Periasamy, A., Haq, Q.M.I. and Malathi, V.G. (2008) An improved DNA isolation method and PCR protocol for efficient detection of multicomponents of begomovirus in legumes. *Journal of Virological Methods*, **147**, 37–42.

42. Tsai, Y.L. and Olson, B.H. (1992) Detection of low numbers of bacterial-cells in soils and sediments by polymerase chain-reaction. *Applied and Environmental Microbiology*, **58**, 754–757.

43. Watson, R.J. and Blackwell, B. (2000) Purification and characterization of a common soil component which inhibits the polymerase chain reaction. *Canadian Journal of Microbiology*, **46**, 633–642.

44. Kermekchiev, M.B., Kirilova, L.I., Vail, E.E. and Barnes, W.M. (2009) Mutants of Taq DNA polymerase resistant to PCR inhibitors allow DNA amplification from whole blood and crude soil samples. *Nucleic Acids Research*, **37**, e40.

45. Khan, G., Kangro, H.O., Coates, P.J. and Heath, R.B. (1991) Inhibitory effects of urine on the polymerase chain-reaction for cytomegalovirus DNA. *Journal of Clinical Pathology*, **44**, 360–365.

46. Abu Al-Soud, W. and Radstrom, P. (1998) Capacity of nine thermostable DNA polymerases to mediate DNA amplification in the presence of PCR-Inhibiting samples. *Applied and Environmental Microbiology*, **64**, 3748–3753.

47. Lantz, P.G., Abu al-Soud, W., Knutsson, R., Hahn-Hagerdal, B. and Radstrom, P. (2000) Biotechnical use of polymerase chain reaction for microbiological analysis of biological samples. *Biotechnology Annual Review*, **5**, 87–130.

48. Eckhart, L., Bach, J., Ban, J. and Tschachler, E. (2000) Melanin binds reversibly to thermostable DNA polymerase and inhibits its activity. *Biochemical and Biophysical Research Communications*, **271**, 726–730.

49. Larkin, A. and Harbison, S.A. (1999) An improved method for STR analysis of bloodstained denim. *International Journal of Legal Medicine*, **112**, 388–390.

50. Kim, S., Labbe, R.G. and Ryu, S. (2000) Inhibitory effects of collagen on the PCR for detection of Clostridium perfringens. *Applied and Environmental Microbiology*, **66**, 1213–1215.

51. Kontanis, E.J. and Reed, F.A. (2006) Evaluation of real-time PCR amplification efficiencies to detect PCR inhibitors. *Journal of Forensic Science*, **51**, 795–804.

52. Port, N.J., Bowyer, V.I., Graham, E.A., Batuwangala, M.S., Rutty, G.N. (2006) How long does it take a static speaking individual to contaminate the immediate environment. *Forensic Science Medicine and Pathology*, **2**, 157–164.

53. Rutty, G.N., Hopwood, A. and Tucker, V. (2003) The effectiveness of protective clothing in the reduction of potential DNA contamination of the scene of crime. *International Journal of Legal Medicine*, **117**, 170–174.

6 The analysis of short tandem repeats

STRs were first used in forensic casework in the early 1990s [1–3]. By the end of the decade they had become the standard tool for just about every forensic laboratory in the world. Today the vast majority of forensic genetic casework involves the analysis of STR polymorphisms and this situation is unlikely to change in the near future [4].

Structure of STR loci

STRs contain a core repeat region between 1 bp[1] and 6 bp long and have alleles that are generally less than 350 bp long. A large number of STR loci have been characterized [5] but only around 20 are commonly analysed in forensic casework (Table 6.1).

The STRs that are widely used in forensic genetics have either a 4 bp or 5 bp core-repeat motif and can be classified as a simple repeat, simple repeat with non-consensus repeats, compound repeat or complex repeat [6] (Figure 6.1).

The development of STR multiplexes

The forensic community has selected STR loci to incorporate into multiplex reactions based on several features including:

- discrete and distinguishable alleles;
- amplification of the locus should be robust;
- a high power of discrimination;
- an absence of genetic linkage with other loci being analysed;
- low levels of artefact formation during the amplification (see Chapter 7);
- the ability to be amplified as part of a multiplex PCR.

---

[1] Note: STRs with repeating core units of 1 bp are not used in forensic analysis.

An Introduction to Forensic Genetics Second Edition   William Goodwin, Adrian Linacre and Sibte Hadi
© 2011 John Wiley & Sons, Ltd

Table 6.1 The development of STR systems. Two STR systems, the quadruplex (QUAD) and SGM were developed by the Forensic Science Service in the UK. The AmpF𝓁STR® SGM Plus® became commercially available in 1998 and has been adopted by a large number of laboratories for routine forensic casework. The AmpF𝓁STR® Identifiler® and PowerPlex® 16 both analyse 15 STR including the 13 loci CODIS loci that are required to be analysed for forensic casework in the USA. The two kits are used widely worldwide, particularly for kinship testing; other kits with additional loci are also available (see Chapter 10)

QUAD	SGM	SGM Plus®	Identifiler®	PowerPlex® 16
vWA	Amelogenin	Amelogenin	Amelogenin	Amelogenin
TH01	vWA	D3S1358	D3S1358	D3S1358
F13A1	D8S1179	vWA	vWA	vWA
FES	D21S11	D16S359	D16S359	D16S359
	D18S51	D8S1179	D8S1179	D8S1179
	TH01	D21S11	D21S11	D21S11
	FGA	D18S51	D18S51	D18S51
		TH01	TH01	TH01
		FGA	FGA	FGA
			D13S317	D13S317
			CSF1PO	CSF1PO
			D7S820	D7S820
			TPOX	TPOX
			D5S818	D5S818
		D2S1338	D2S1338	Penta D
		D19S433	D19S433	Penta E

TH01 – Simple repeat with a non-consensus allele

| AATG | AATG | AATG | AATG | AATG | AATG | AATG | allele 7

| AATG | AATG | AATG | AATG | AATG | AATG | ATG | AATG | AATG | AATG | allele 9.3

FGA – Compound repeat

allele 17

allele 20

☐ TTTC   ■ TTTT   ▨ TTCT   ☐ CTTT   ▨ CTCC   ■ TTCC

D21S11 – Complex repeat sequence

allele 28

allele 30.2

☐ TCTA   ■ TCTG   ▮ TA   ☐ Sequence not included in repeat

Figure 6.1 The structure of three commonly used STR loci, TH01, FGA and D21S11. The TH01 locus has a simple repeat with a non-consensus allele; in the example, the 9.3 allele is missing the first A from the seventh repeat. The FGA locus is a compound repeat composed of several elements. The D21S11 allele is an example of a complex repeat; the three regions not included in the FGA nomenclature are an invariant TA, TCA and TCCATA sequence

An essential feature of any STR used in forensic analysis is that biological material should give an identical profile regardless of the individual or laboratory that carries out the analysis. Without this standardization it would not be possible to compare results between laboratories, and developments such as national DNA databases would not be possible [7–11]. All new multiplexes have to be vigorously validated before they are used for the analysis of casework [12–20].

The UK Forensic Science Service (FSS) developed the first STR-based typing system that was designed for forensic analysis in 1994. Four STR loci were amplified in the same reaction [16, 21, 22]. This was replaced by the second generation multiplex (SGM), which was also developed by the FSS [23–25]. With the increased adoption of STR multiplexes worldwide, two commercial companies, Applied Biosystems and Promega Corporation, have developed a series of multiplexes that are now used by most laboratories. The AmpFℓSTR® SGM Plus, which is produced by Applied Biosystems replaced the SGM in the UK and has been adopted by many other countries around the world as one of their standard multiplex kits [12]. In the USA, STR technology was adopted into forensic casework following a survey of 17 previously characterized STR loci, and in 1997 13 loci were selected as the Combined DNA Index System (CODIS) loci [8, 26]. These loci can be analysed in one PCR using one of two commercially available kits; the AmpFℓSTR® Identifiler® produced by Applied Biosystems [27] and the PowerPlex® 16 produced by Promega Corporation [14]. Additional commercial kits are available that incorporate additional loci, for example the SinoFiler™, which has been designed for the Chinese market, and replaces four of the loci found in the Identifiler® [28]. The STR loci that are incorporated into some commonly used multiplexes are shown in Table 6.1.

In addition to STR loci, the amelogenin locus, which is present on the X and Y, chromosomes has been incorporated into all commonly used STR multiplex kits. The amelogenin gene encodes for a protein that is a major component of tooth enamel matrix; there are two versions of the gene, the copy on the X chromosome has a 6 bp deletion, and this length polymorphism allows the versions of the gene on the X and Y chromosomes to be differentiated [29] (Figure 6.2).

Figure 6.2 The amelogenin locus is present on both the X and Y chromosomes. The gene that is present on the X chromosome has a 6 bp deletion. The primers (schematically shown by the arrowed lines) that were reported by Sullivan et al. [29] led to products of 106 bp from the X chromosome and 112 bp from the Y chromosome

Detection of STR polymorphisms

After STR polymorphisms have been amplified using PCR, the length of the products must be measured precisely – some STR alleles differ by only 1 bp. Gel electrophoresis of the PCR products through denaturing polyacrylamide gels can be used to separate DNA molecules between 20 and 500 nucleotides long with single base pair resolution [30]. Early systems detected the PCR products after electrophoresis on polyacrylamide slab-gels using silver staining [31, 32], but this limited the number of loci that could be incorporated into the multiplexes because the allelic size ranges of the different loci could not overlap. To overcome this limitation, fluorescence labelling of PCR products followed by multicolour detection has been adopted by the forensic community. A series of fluorescent dyes has been developed that can be covalently attached to the 5′ end of one of the PCR primers in each primer pair and detected real-time during electrophoresis. Up to five different dyes can be used in a single analysis, which allows for considerable overlap of loci (Figure 6.3). The electrophoresis platforms have evolved from systems based on slab-gels to capillary electrophoresis (CE), which use a narrow glass tube filled with an entangled polymer

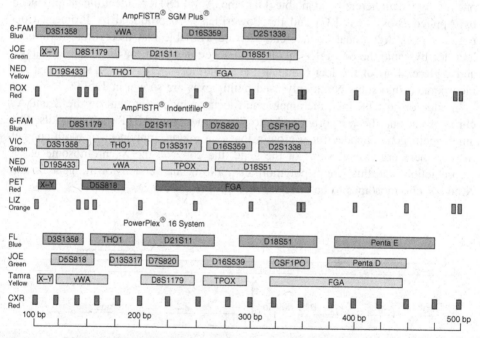

Figure 6.3 PCR multiplexes use up to five different dyes to label PCR products. The allelic ranges of three commonly used multiplexes, the AmpFℓSTR® SGM Plus®, AmpFℓSTR® Identifiler® and the PowerPlex® 16 are shown. The use of multiple dyes allows the detection of the internal-lane size standard (ROX™ in SGM Plus, LIZ™ in Identifiler® and CXR in PowerPlex® 16) and three or four overlapping STR loci, where the use of different dyes allows the alleles to be assigned to the correct locus

solution to separate the DNA molecules [33–37]. Applied Biosystems provide the most commonly used CE systems and all these have multicolour detection capacity. The ABI PRISM® 310 Genetic Analyzer has a single capillary and analyses up to 48 samples per day; the ABI PRISM® 3100, 3130*xl* and 3500 Genetic Analyzers, which have up to 16 capillaries and can analyse over 1000 samples per day, and the ABI PRISM® 3700 and Applied Biosystems 3730*xl* Genetic Analyzers, which can have up to 96 capillaries and can analyse over 4000 samples per day.

Before electrophoresis, the PCR sample is prepared by mixing approximately 1 µl of the reaction with 10–20 µl of deionized formamide. The internal-lane size standard is also added at this point. The deionized formamide denatures the DNA; heating the samples to 95 °C is routinely carried out to ensure that the PCR products are single-stranded. The samples are transferred into the capillary using electrokinetic injection, a voltage is applied and charged molecules, including the amplified DNA fragments and the internal lane size standards, migrate into the capillary. After injection, a constant voltage is applied across the capillary and the PCR products migrate towards the positively charged anode, travelling through the polymer that fills the capillary and acts as the sieving matrix. Urea and 2-pyrrolidinone in the gel polymer and a temperature of 60 °C help to prevent the formation of any secondary structure during electrophoresis [38]. Throughout the period of electrophoresis, an argon ion laser is shone through a small glass window in the capillary, and as PCR products labelled with fluorescent dyes travel past the window they are excited by the laser and emit fluorescence, which is detected by a charged coupled device (CCD) camera, and then are recorded by collection software [39] (Figure 6.4). The electrophoresis of a sample takes up to 30 minutes after which the

Figure 6.4 During electrophoresis an argon laser is shone through the window in the capillary. As the labelled PCR products migrate through the gel towards the anode they are separated based on their size. When the laser hits the fluorescent label on the PCR products it is excited and emits fluorescent light which passes though a filter to remove any background noise and then onto a charged coupled device camera that detects the wavelength of the light and sends the information to a computer where software records the profile

polymer in the capillary is replaced with fresh polymer and the next sample can be analysed.

Interpretation of STR profiles

The spectra of the dyes used to label the PCR products overlap and the raw data contain peaks that are composed of more than one dye colour. After data collection the GeneScan® or GeneMapper™ *ID* software removes spectral overlap in the profile and calculates the sizes of the amplified DNA fragments. The software calculates how much spectral overlap there is between each dye and subtracts this from the peaks within the profile (Figure 6.5). A good matrix file, which contains information on the amount of overlap in the spectra, will produce peaks within the profile that are composed of only one colour. The height of the peaks is measured in relative fluorescent units (RFU); the height is proportional to the amount of PCR product that is detected.

To be able to size the PCR products an internal-lane size standard is used. The internal-lane size standards contain fragments of DNA of known length that are labelled with a fluorescent dye, and the fragments are detected along with the amplified PCR products during CE [40]. Commonly used commercial internal-lane size standards are the GeneScan™-500 standards that can be labelled with either ROX™ or LIZ™ dyes (Applied Biosystems) and the ILS600 (Promega Corporation) (Figure 6.6).

(a)

(b)

Figure 6.5 The application of a matrix file, using the GeneScan® or GeneMapperID® software removes the spectral overlap from the raw data (a) to produce peaks within the profile that are composed of only one colour (b)

Figure 6.6 Internal-lane size standards are used to precisely size the PCR products. Two commonly used internal-lane size standards are (a) the GeneScan™-500 (Applied Biosystems) and (b) the ILS600 (Promega Corporation)

Because the internal-lane size standard is analysed along with each PCR, any differences between runs that could affect the migration rates during electrophoresis, such as temperature, do not impact significantly on the analysis [41]. The software generates a size calling curve from the internal-lane size standards; the data point of the unknown fragments are compared with the size calling curve. Different algorithms have been developed to measure the size of DNA molecules, the most common one is the local Southern method [42] (Figure 6.7).

After analysing the raw data with the software the end result is an electropherogram with a series of peaks that represent different alleles: the size, peak height and peak area is also measured by the software (Figure 6.8). The final stage of generating a STR profile is to assign specific alleles to the amplified PCR products. Each peak in the profile is given a number that is a description of the structure of that allele; this is straightforward when naming simple repeats but is more problematic with complex repeat sequences [6].

The loci used in forensic casework have been well characterized and multiple alleles have been sequenced to determine the allelic structure and verify that the size of the peaks is a good indicator of the alleles they represent. However, because the migration of PCR products and internal-lane size standard varies slightly with factors such as temperature and the electrophoretic conditions, and because some STR alleles

(a)   (b)

Figure 6.7 During electrophoresis the computer software records the fluorescence levels at regular time points and these are recorded as data points. The DNA fragments that make up the internal-lane size standards are plotted against the data points. An example of the sizing curves that are produced from (a) the GeneScan®-500 standard (Applied Biosystems) and (b) the ILS600 (Promega Corporation) are shown using the local Southern method to generate the size calling curve

Dye/Sample Peak	Minutes	Size	Peak Height	Peak Area	Data Point	
8G, 24	13.13	103.33	4058	20712	3579	} amelogenin
8G, 29	13.32	109.01	4017	20507	3633	
8G, 46	14.22	135.89	2784	17224	3877	} D8S1179
8G, 51	14.49	144.74	3550	19959	3950	
8G, 89	16.50	208.66	2820	17157	4499	} D21S11
8G, 92	16.69	214.59	3310	20136	4550	
8G, 135	19.00	290.90	2159	16332	5180	} D18S51
8G, 136	19.12	295.06	2144	16104	5213	

Figure 6.8 The green loci from a profile produced using the AmpF*ℓ*STR® SGM Plus® kit. The size of each peak has been calculated along with the peak heights and areas. The first amelogenin peak was detected after 13.13 minutes (which is when data point 3579 was taken) and is estimated to be 103.33 bp long, the peak area is 20 712 rfu and the peak height 4058 rfu

differ by only 1 bp, the use of allelic ladders that contain all the common alleles (Figure 6.9) at each locus has been adopted by the forensic community to ensure accurate profiling [16, 43]. Unlike the internal-lane size standards the allelic ladders cannot be analysed in the same injection as the samples, but are run periodically during the analysis of a batch of samples.

When assigning the alleles, the unknown peaks are compared with the allelic ladder and should fall within a 1-bp window, that is ±0.5 bp of the allelic ladder size; if the unknown alleles differ by more than this then they are classified as off-ladder (OL)

Figure 6.9 The allelic ladder of the AmpFℓSTR® SGM Plus® kit contains all the common alleles

Figure 6.10 The comparison of an unknown allele with the allelic ladder allows the THO1 alleles to be classified as 7 and 9.3. The size of the unknown allele and the allele in the allelic ladder are not identical but fall within 0.5 bp of each other. The 0.5 bp match windows are indicated by the shaded areas

and require further analysis. This comparison of unknown peaks to the allelic ladder can be done manually or by using the Genotyper® (Figure 6.10) or GeneMapper™ *ID* software (Applied Biosystems), which will compare all the unknown alleles in the profile to the allelic ladder.

The final result is a profile where alleles have been assigned to all of the peaks in the profile (Figure 6.11).

The STR profiles should generate the same allele designations regardless of the laboratory where the analysis took place or the variations in the methodology that may

Figure 6.11 The Genotyper® software compares the peaks within a profile to the allelic ladder and assigns alleles. If the peaks in the profile deviate more than ±0.5 bp from the allelic ladder they are designates 'off ladder'

Table 6.2 Profiles have been generated from the same DNA sample using three commercial kits, the AmpF*l*STR® SGM Plus®, AmpF*l*STR® Identifiler® and the PowerPlex® 16. The alleles that are detected in the loci that are common between the kits are all identical

Locus	Profile					
	SGM Plus®		Identifiler®		PowerPlex® 16	
Amelogenin	X	Y	X	Y	X	Y
D3S1358	15	17	15	17	15	17
vWA	14	17	14	17	14	17
D16S359	11	13	11	13	11	13
D8S1179	11	13	11	13	11	13
D21S11	30	31.2	30	31.2	30	31.2
D18S51	14	15	14	15	14	15
TH01	9	9.3	9	9.3	9	9.3
FGA	21	21	21	21	21	21
D13S317	–	–	10	14	10	14
CSF1PO	–	–	9	12	9	12
D7S820	–	–	8	10	8	10
TPOX	–	–	11	11	11	11
D5S818	–	–	11	13	11	13
D2S1338	24	25	24	25	–	–
D19S433	14	15.2	14	15.2	–	–
Penta D	–	–	–	–	12	13
Penta E	–	–	–	–	12	14

have been used to generate the profile, such as different DNA extraction and quantification techniques and CE platforms. Loci that are included in different commercial kits should also produce identical results (Table 6.2).

Further reading

Butler, J.M. (2005) *Forensic DNA Typing: Biology, Technology and Genetics of STR Markers*, 2nd edn, Academic Press, London.
Butler, J.M. (2006) Genetics and genomics of core short tandem repeat loci used in human identity testing. *Journal of Forensic Sciences* **51**, 253–265.

WWW resource

Ruitberg, C.M., Reeder, D.J. and Butler, J.M. (2001) STRBase: a short tandem repeat DNA database for the human identity testing community. *Nucleic Acids Research* **29**, 320–322. http://www.cstl.nist.gov/div831/strbase/.

References

1. Clayton, T.M., Whitaker, J.P. and Maguire, C.N. (1995) Identification of bodies from the scene of a mass disaster using DNA amplification of short tandem repeat (STR) loci. *Forensic Science International*, **76**, 7–15.
2. Hagelberg, E., Gray, I.C. and Jeffreys, A.J. (1991) Identification of the skeletal remains of a murder victim by DNA analysis. *Nature*, **352**, 427–429.
3. Jeffreys, A.J., Allen, M.J., Hagelberg, E. and Sonnberg, A. (1992) Identification of the skeletal remains of Josef Mengele by DNA analysis. *Forensic Science International*, **56**, 65–76.
4. Gill, P., Werrett, D.J., Budowle, B. and Guerrieri, R. (2004) An assessment of whether SNPs will replace STRs in national DNA databases. *Science and Justice*, **44**, 51–53.
5. Ruitberg, C.M., Reeder, D.J. and Butler, J.M. (2001) STRBase: a short tandem repeat DNA database for the human identity testing community. *Nucleic Acids Research*, **29**, 320–322.
6. Gill, P., Brinkmann, B., d'Aloja, E., Andersen, J., Bar, W. and Carracedo, A. *et al.* (1997) Considerations from the European DNA profiling group (EDNAP) concerning STR nomenclature. *Forensic Science International*, **87**, 185–192.
7. Andersen, J., Martin, P., Carracedo, A., Dobosz, M., Eriksen, B., Johnsson, V. *et al.* (1996) Report on the third EDNAP collaborative STR exercise. *Forensic Science International*, **78**, 83–93.
8. Budowle, B., Moretti, T.R., Niezgoda, S.J. and Brown, B.L. (eds) (1998) CODIS and PCR-based short tandem repeat loci: law enforcement tools. Second European Symposium on Human Identification, Promega Corporation, pp. 73–88.
9. Gill, P., d'Aloja, E., Andersen, J., Dupuy, B., Jangblad, M., Johnsson, V. *et al.* (1997) Report of the European DNA profiling group (EDNAP): an investigation of the complex STR loci D21S11 and HUMFIBRA (FGA). *Forensic Science International*, **86**, 25–33.
10. Gill, P., Kimpton, C., Daloja, E., Andersen, J.F., Bar, W., Brinkmann, B. *et al.* (1994) Report of the European DNA Profiling Group (EDNAP) – towards standardization of short tandem repeat (STR) loci. *Forensic Science International*, **65**, 51–59.
11. Gill, P., Sparkes, R., Fereday, L. and Werrett, D.J. (2000) Report of the European Network of Forensic Science Institutes (ENSFI): formulation and testing of principles to evaluate STR multiplexes. *Forensic Science International*, **108**, 1–29.
12. Cotton, E.A., Allsop, R.F., Guest, J.L., Frazier, R.R.E., Koumi, P., Callow, I.P. *et al.* (2000) Validation of the AmpFℓSTR (R) SGM Plus (TM) system for use in forensic casework. *Forensic Science International*, **112**, 151–161.

13. Fregeau, C.J., Brown, K.L., Leclair, B., Trudel, I., Bishop, L. and Fourney, R.M. (2003) AmpF*l*STR (R) Profiler Plus (TM) short tandem repeat DNA analysis of casework samples, mixture samples, and nonhuman DNA samples amplified under reduced PCR volume conditions (25 mu L). *Journal of Forensic Sciences*, **48**, 1014–1034.

14. Krenke, B.E., Tereba, A., Anderson, S.J., Buel, E., Culhane, S., Finis, C.J. *et al.* (2002) Validation of a 16-locus fluorescent multiplex system. *Journal of Forensic Sciences*, **47**, 773–785.

15. LaFountain, M.J., Schwartz, M.B., Svete, P.A., Walkinshaw, M.A. and Buel, E. (2001) TWGDAM validation of the AmpF*l*STR Profiler Plus and AmpF*l*STR COfiler STR multiplex systems using capillary electrophoresis. *Journal of Forensic Sciences*, **46**, 1191–1198.

16. Lygo, J.E., Johnson, P.E., Holdaway, D.J., Woodroffe, S., Whitaker, J.P., Clayton, T.M. *et al.* (1994) The validation of short tandem repeat (STR) loci for use in forensic casework. *International Journal of Legal Medicine*, **107**, 77–89.

17. Moretti, T.R., Baumstark, A.L., Defenbaugh, D.A., Keys, K.M., Brown, A.L. and Budowle, B. (2001) Validation of STR typing by capillary electrophoresis. *Journal of Forensic Sciences*, **46**, 661–676.

18. Moretti, T.R., Baumstark, A.L., Defenbaugh, D.A., Keys, K.M., Smerick, J.B. and Budowle, B. (2001) Validation of short tandem repeats (STRs) for forensic usage: Performance testing of fluorescent multiplex STR systems and analysis of authentic and simulated forensic samples. *Journal of Forensic Sciences*, **46**, 647–660.

19. Thomson, J.A., Pilotti, V., Stevens, P., Ayres, K.L. and Debenham, P.G. (1999) Validation of short tandem repeat analysis for the investigation of cases of disputed paternity. *Forensic Science International*, **100**, 1–16.

20. Wallin, J.M., Buoncristiani, M.R., Lazaruk, K.D., Fildes, N., Holt, C.L. and Walsh, P.S. (1998) TWGDAM validation of the AmpFISTR (TM) Blue PCR amplification kit for forensic casework analysis. *Journal of Forensic Sciences*, **43**, 854–870.

21. Clayton, T.M., Whitaker, J.P., Fisher, D.L., Lee, D.A., Holland, M.M., Weedn, V.W. *et al.* (1995) Further validation of a quadruplex STR DNA typing system: a collaborative effort to identify victims of a mass disaster. *Forensic Science International*, **76**, 17–25.

22. Kimpton, C., Fisher, D., Watson, S., Adams, M., Urquhart, A., Lygo, J. *et al.* (1994) Evaluation of an automated DNA profiling system employing multiplex amplification of 4 tetrameric STR loci. *International Journal of Legal Medicine*, **106**, 302–311.

23. Kimpton, C.P., Oldroyd, N.J., Watson, S.K., Frazier, R.R.E., Johnson, P.E., Millican, E.S. *et al.* (1996) Validation of highly discriminating multiplex short tandem repeat amplification systems for individual identification. *Electrophoresis*, **17**, 1283–1293.

24. Sparkes, R., Kimpton, C., Gilbard, S., Carne, P., Andersen, J., Oldroyd, N. *et al.* (1996) The validation of a 7-locus multiplex STR test for use in forensic casework. 2. Artefacts, casework studies and success rates. *International Journal of Legal Medicine*, **109**, 195–204.

25. Sparkes, R., Kimpton, C., Watson, S., Oldroyd, N., Clayton, T., Barnett, L. *et al.* (1996) The validation of a 7-locus multiplex STR test for use in forensic casework. 1. Mixtures, ageing, degradation and species studies. *International Journal of Legal Medicine*, **109**, 186–194.

26. Budowle, B., Moretti, T.R., Baumstark, A.L., Defenbaugh, D.A., Keys, K.M. *et al.* (1999) Population data on the thirteen CODIS core short tandem repeat loci in African Americans, US Caucasians, Hispanics, Bahamians, Jamaicans, and Trinidadians. *Journal of Forensic Sciences*, **44**, 1277–1286.

27. Collins, P.J., Hennessy, L.K., Leibelt, C.S., Roby, R.K., Reeder, D.J. and Foxall, P.A. (2004) Developmental validation of a single-tube amplification of the 13 CODIS STR loci, D2S1338, D19S433, and amelogenin: the AmpF*l*STR (R) Identifiler (R) PCR amplification kit. *Journal of Forensic Sciences*, **49**, 1265–1277.

28. Huang, S., Zhu, Y., Shen, X., Le, X. and Yan, H. (2010) Genetic variation analysis of 15 autosomal STR loci of AmpF'STR Sinofiler™ PCR Amplification Kit in Henan (central China) Han population. *Legal Medicine*, **12**, 160–161.

29. Sullivan, K.M., Mannucci, A., Kimpton, C.P. and Gill, P. (1993) A rapid and quantitative DNA sex test – fluorescence-based PCR analysis of X-Y homologous gene amelogenin. *Biotechniques*, **15**, 636–638.

30. Ziegle, J.S., Su, Y., Corcoran, K.P., Nie, L., Mayrand, P.E., Hoff, L.B. *et al.* (1992) Application of automated DNA sizing technology for genotyping microsatellite loci. *Genomics*, **14**, 1026–1031.

31. Lins, A.M., Sprecher, C.J., Puers, C. and Schumm, J.W. (1996) Multiplex sets for the amplification of polymorphic short tandem repeat loci – silver stain and fluorescence detection. *Biotechniques*, **20**, 882–889.

32. Sprecher, C.J., Puers, C., Lins, A.M. and Schumm, J.W. (1996) General approach to analysis of polymorphic short tandem repeat loci. *Biotechniques*, **20**, 266–267.

33. Buel, E., Schwartz, M.B. and LaFountain, M.J. (1998) Capillary electrophoresis STR analysis: comparison to Gel-based systems. *Journal of Forensic Sciences*, **43**, 164–170.

34. Butler, J.M., Buel, E., Crivellente, F. and McCord, B.R. (2004) Forensic DNA typing by capillary electrophoresis using the ABI Prism 310 and 3100 genetic analyzers for STR analysis. *Electrophoresis*, **25**, 1397–1412.

35. Butler, J.M., McCord, B.R., Jung, J.M., Lee, J.A., Budowle, B. and Allen, R.O. (1995) Application of dual internal standards for precise sizing of polymerase chain-reaction products using capillary electrophoresis. *Electrophoresis*, **16**, 974–980.

36. Heiger, D.N., Cohen, A.S. and Karger, B.L. (1990) Separation of DNA restriction fragments by high-performance capillary electrophoresis with low and zero cross-linked polyacrylamide using continuous and pulsed electric-fields. *Journal of Chromatography*, **516**, 33–48.

37. Madabhushi, R.S. (1998) Separation of 4-color DNA sequencing extension products in noncovalently coated capillaries using low viscosity polymer solutions. *Electrophoresis*, **19**, 224–230.

38. Rosenblum, B.B., Oaks, F., Menchen, S. and Johnson, B. (1997) Improved single-strand DNA sizing accuracy in capillary electrophoresis. *Nucleic Acids Research*, **25**, 3925–3929.

39. Butler, J. (2001) *Forensic DNA Typing: Biology and Technology Behind STR Markers*, Academic Press.

40. Edwards, A., Civitello, A., Hammond, H.A. and Caskey, C.T. (1991) DNA typing and genetic-mapping with trimeric and tetrameric tandem repeats. *American Journal of Human Genetics*, **49**, 746–756.

41. Hartzell, B., Graham, K. and McCord, B. (2003) Response of short tandem repeat systems to temperature and sizing methods. *Forensic Science International*, **133**, 228–234.

42. Elder, J.K. and Southern, E.M. (1983) Measurement of DNA length by gel-electrophoresis 2. Comparison of methods for relating mobility to fragment length. *Analytical Biochemistry*, **128**, 227–231.

43. Smith, R.N. (1995) Accurate size comparison of short tandem repeat alleles amplified by PCR. *Biotechniques*, **18**, 122–128.

7 Assessment of STR profiles

DNA profiles generated from casework samples require some experience to interpret. Guidelines have evolved to assist with the interpretation of STR profiles, ensuring that the results are robust and consistent; this is especially important when dealing with samples that contain very small amounts of DNA, degraded DNA or mixtures of profiles that come from two or more individuals – all situations that complicate interpretation. This chapter explores a number of artefacts that can occur in DNA profiles. Some casework scenarios that can lead to complex profiles are also considered.

Stutter peaks

During the amplification of an STR allele it is normal to generate a stutter peak, that is one repeat unit smaller or larger that the true allele; smaller alleles are formed in the majority of cases [1]. Stutter peaks are formed by strand slippage during the extension of the nascent DNA strand during PCR amplification (Figure 7.1) [2, 3].

Even in good-quality profiles there will be some stutter peaks; these are recognizable and do not interfere with the interpretation of the profile. Threshold limits are normally used to aid in the identification and interpretation of stutter peaks, so, for example although the degree of stutter varies between loci, they are typically less than 15% of the main peak [4, 5]; understanding stutter peaks is especially important when interpreting mixtures.

Different STR loci have varying tendencies to stutter. This is dependent on the structure of the core repeats: di- and trinucleotide repeats are more prone to stutter than are tetra- and pentanucleotide repeats, and this is one of the reasons that all the autosomal STRs that have been adopted by the forensic community have tetra- and pentanucleotide core repeats (Figure 7.2). STRs with simple core repeats tend to have higher stutter rates than compound and complex repeats.

Split peaks (±N)

The *Taq* polymerase that is used to drive the PCR adds nucleotides to the newly synthesized DNA molecule in a template-dependent manner.

However, it also has an activity, called terminal transferase, whereby it adds a nucleotide to the end of the amplified molecule which is non-template-dependent [6]. Approximately 85% of the time an adenine residue is added (Figure 7.3).

An Introduction to Forensic Genetics Second Edition   William Goodwin, Adrian Linacre and Sibte Hadi
© 2011 John Wiley & Sons, Ltd

Figure 7.1 During PCR slippage between the template and the nascent DNA strands leads to the copied strand containing one repeat less than the template strand

Figure 7.2 Stutter peaks are formed during slippage of the *Taq* polymerase during replication of the template strand. The slippage results in amplification products one repeat unit shorter than the template. The stutter peaks are normally less than 15% of the true amplification product. (a) A dinucleotide repeat which is prone to high levels of slippage; the stutter peaks are indicated by the arrow and their size relative to the main peak is shown (based on peak area). (b) A tetranucleotide repeat which displays lower levels of stutter

Figure 7.3 The *Taq* polymerase adds a nucleotide to the 3′ end of the newly synthesized strand. The non-template addition is usually an adenine and results in a PCR product that is 1 bp longer than the template (N + 1). The arrowed lines represent the forward and reverse primers

Figure 7.4 Split peaks are seen in profiles when the non-template addition does not occur with all of the PCR products. The three examples show decreasing amounts of non-template addition with (a) showing an example where the vast majority of PCR product has the non-template addition, (b) with around 25% non-template addition through to (c) where only 50% of the PCR product has the non-template addition

It is important that the vast majority of PCR products have the non-template nucleotide added, otherwise a split peak is observed in the DNA profile (Figure 7.4). Split peaks are usually caused either by the suboptimal activity of the *Taq* polymerase or by too much template DNA in the PCR.

In order to minimize the formation of split peaks in a profile, at the end of the cycling stage of the PCR, the reaction is incubated at 65 °C–72 °C for between 45 and 60 minutes, allowing the *Taq* polymerase to complete the non-template addition of all the PCR products.

The interpretation of profiles with split peaks is possible because the peak with the nucleotide added is taken as being the correct peak. Problems can occur when alleles are present that differ by only 1 bp; the TH01 9.3 allele, for example, could be confused with the TH01 allele 10. In most cases, a profile with a high degree of split peaks would have to be re-analysed to minimize the possibility of incorrect interpretation.

Pull-up

In Chapter 6 the matrix file was introduced; this file contains information about the levels of spectral overlap that exist with the dyes that have been used to label the PCR products. This information is used by the Genescan® and GeneMapper™ *ID* software to produce peaks that are made up of one colour. If the matrix file is not of good quality then this correction is not perfect and the peaks in the resulting profile are composed of more than one colour; this phenomenon is called pull-up. Pull-ups are easy to recognize as a smaller product will appear at exactly the same size as the real STR allele. Pull-up can also occur when there has been over-amplification, even if the matrix file is of good quality (Figure 7.5a).

Figure 7.5 If the reaction is overloaded with DNA (a) the peaks are still present but artefacts such as pull-ups and split peaks are more pronounced. When the template is within the optimal range (b and c) the peaks are well balanced and easy to interpret. When the PCR does not have enough template to amplify (d) then locus and allelic drop-out can occur

Template DNA

Commercial STR kits have been optimized to amplify small amounts of template DNA, commonly between 0.5 ng and 2.5 ng, which represents approximately 166 and 833 copies of the haploid human genome. It is not always possible to add the optimum amount of DNA to a PCR when the sample size is limited.

Overloaded profiles

Overloading the PCR can also lead to a profile that is difficult to interpret. If the CCD camera is saturated, then the peak height/area is no longer a good indicator of the amount of product and this can lead to problems in assessing peak balance and can make the interpretation of mixtures difficult. Overloaded profiles also tend to have a noisy baseline, increased levels of stuttering, split peaks and pull-ups (Figure 7.6).

Low template DNA typing

At many crime scenes it may be possible to infer surfaces with which the perpetrator has had physical contact, for example the handle of a gun, a knife, a ligature, a door handle or a steering wheel. These areas can be swabbed to collect any epithelial cells that have been shed during the contact [6–9]. The amounts of DNA extracted can be extremely low but in some circumstances it is possible to get a full DNA profile from less than 100 pg of template DNA: the normal range of template DNA is between 500 pg and 2500 pg (2.5 ng). To analyse such small quantities of DNA the

Figure 7.6 A heavily overloaded profile. All the peaks shown have a flat top, indicating that they are off-scale, the baseline is very noisy, several split peaks are evident and the peaks are very broad which can lead to sizing problems. There are also some pronounced stutter peaks

number of amplification cycles is increased to 34, termed low copy number (LCN) when introduced by the Forensic Science Service, UK. The standard number of cycles in the amplification using commercial kits is between 28 and 32 cycles. Empirical studies have shown that above 34 cycles the amount of artefacts that are detected outweigh the benefit of higher levels of artefact [10]. Extreme care has to be taken when interpreting LCN profiles (low template number) [10, 11]. A number of features can be seen when amplifying low amounts of template DNA. These are allele drop-out and drop-in; severe peak imbalance; locus drop-out (Figure 7.5d); and increased stutter [11–13]. Allele drop-out occurs when through chance events one allele in a heterozygous locus is preferentially amplified; this can give the false impression that the profile at a particular locus is homozygous. PCR must be repeated at least twice to minimize the possibility of this occurring and only alleles that appear in two or more amplifications can be called (Figure 7.7).

This phenomenon also leads to a peak imbalance that is much higher than when using higher amounts of template DNA. Allele drop-in is also a common phenomenon when amplifying low amounts of template DNA. The drop-in alleles are spurious amplification products from unknown DNA, such as cells from operators and on plasticware. As allele drop-in is a random event; it is unlikely that the same allele will be amplified in both samples of a duplicate or triplicate reactions, but they can still confuse the interpretation of the profile. Locus drop-out, particularly of the larger

Figure 7.7 Three separate PCR analyses of a DNA extract can lead to different results. When dealing with very low template numbers allelic drop-out is relatively common and the true genotype can only be ascertained through multiple amplifications; even then the results can be contentious

STR loci, can also occur; this reduces the amount of information from the profile but does not confuse the interpretation. At present, there is no clear consensus in the scientific community about the use of LCN PCR [14]. LCN was prominent in the trial of the one person accused of involvement with the Omagh bombing in 1998. Although the process was supported by a Home Office inquiry [15] and is now used in many countries, there remain jurisdictions, including most states in the USA, which prefer to remain with standard cycling conditions and no further enhancements.

Peak balance

STR loci that are used in forensic analysis are commonly heterozygous, producing two peaks in the profile. In a perfect profile the two peaks that are produced are balanced 1:1 in terms of peak height and area, but in reality this is very rare and one peak will be larger than the other (Figure 7.8). The variations in peak height can be due to chance events, where one allele is more efficiently amplified than another. In good-quality DNA extracts, the smaller peak is, on average, approximately 90% the size of the larger peak [5].

Laboratories will use different values that are based on their own validation studies but commonly require the smaller peak of a locus to be within 60% of the larger peak [5]. Peak imbalance can be more extreme when profiling degraded DNA and when amplifying low amounts of template DNA. On rare occasions the mutation of a primer binding site will reduce the efficiency of the PCR for one allele, which can result in high levels of peak imbalance and even allele drop-out. The frequency of these mutations is low, ranging between frequencies of 0.01 and 0.001 per locus [16].

Mixtures

Many biological samples that are recovered from a scene of crime will contain a mixture of cellular material from more than one person. Clothing will often contain cellular material from the wearer and may also contain material from an assailant after an assault; the handle of a door or a steering wheel may have been handled

Figure 7.8 The profile shows the green loci from the SGM Plus® kit. The peak area of the smallest peak at each locus is shown as a percentage of the larger peak. The size of the peaks is proportional to the amount of PCR product; this can be gauged by measuring the peak height or more usually the peak area

Dye/Sample Peak	Minutes	Size	Peak Height	Peak Area	Data Point
G, 20	19.81	286.85	2507	22267	5401
G, 21	20.06	295.47	2322	21374	5470
G, 22	20.18	299.62	981	8673	5503
G, 23	20.67	318.05	904	8285	5636

Figure 7.9 A mixture of two individuals will lead to up to four peaks at each locus. The area between the dotted lines represents the zone where the minor component of the mixture can be interpreted. The dotted lines represent 15% and 60% of the major peaks: below the 15% line is the zone where stutter peaks from the major alleles can occur; peaks below the 60% cannot be easily explained by peak imbalance. At this locus the major component can be interpreted as 13–15 and the minor component's genotype is 16–20

by several people: there are many circumstances when mixtures of material can be collected. A mixture in a DNA profile can be recognized by the presence of more than two alleles at any locus within the profile, normally there will be several loci that have three or four alleles present and a loss of peak balance within individual loci.

Having determined that the profile is mixed, the first task is to assess how many contributors are represented in the profile. Two-person mixtures are most commonly seen in forensic casework; with a two-person mixture a maximum of four alleles will be present at any locus, whereas three-person mixtures will contain up to six alleles at a locus. When four alleles are present at a given locus and there is a major and minor component, the interpretation is relatively simple (Figure 7.9). The ratio of peak areas within a locus generally corresponds with the ratio of template molecules [17–19], peak areas that consider the morphology of the peak as well as the height [16], are commonly used as a guide to interpret mixed profiles [20]. Even in a two-person mixture when there are shared alleles between the major and minor profiles, the interpretation becomes more difficult – especially in mixtures where the minor profile is less than one-third of the level of the major profile [16].

In mixtures where the major component is in large excess, it is often possible to deduce the major profile; however, in such cases it is difficult to get much information from the minor component where the interpretation is complicated by artefacts in the profile, such as stutter peaks, and also by the major profile masking the minor profile [21]. Software has been developed that helps with the interpretation of complex mixtures [22].

Figure 7.10   The SGM Plus® profile appears normal, except for the presence of a third allele at the D16S539 locus

Multiple peaks at one locus

Some STR profiles appear normal, apart from the appearance of an extra allele at one locus (Figure 7.10). In these circumstances it is very unlikely that the third allele is because of a mixture, as we would expect to see three of four alleles at several loci.

The triallelic patterns can be classified into two types: Type 1 patterns contain alleles with different levels of intensity, and occur as a result of a somatic mutation; Type 2 patterns are the result of localized chromosomal rearrangements, resulting in the duplication of the locus, and result in alleles of approximate equal intensity [23–26]. In some rare cases several loci may display more than two alleles [27, 28].

Degraded DNA

Many samples that are collected from a crime scene may have been exposed to the environment for hours, days or even longer if the crime scene has gone undetected. When DNA analysis is being used to identify human remains, the remains may be several years old before they are analysed or may have been exposed to severe environmental insult, such as high temperatures. In all these circumstances the DNA in the cellular material will not be in pristine condition and will have degraded. This leads to a characteristic DNA profile with over-amplification of the smaller loci; the successful amplification declines with the size of the alleles. Figures 7.11 and 7.12 show two examples of degraded DNA sample; the first one is from a bone sample that had been in water for 30 years. The small loci have over-amplified, whereas the

Figure 7.11 The profile was generated using the AmpFℓSTR® Profiler Plus® kit from Applied Biosystems. The DNA was extracted from a bone recovered from a Scottish loch after approximately 30 years. The profile is typical of a degraded profile with a gradual reduction in the amount of product as the amplicons increase in size

Figure 7.12 The profile was generated using the AmpFℓSTR® Blue™ kit from Applied Biosystems. The DNA was extracted from muscle tissue recovered from a plane crash. The muscle had been subjected to high temperatures and the DNA was highly degraded; no amplification products were detected from the FGA locus. The size standard is also shown as the red peaks

larger loci are barely detectable [29]; the decrease in amplification is gradual as the length of the alleles increases.

In the second example an example of locus drop out can be seen, the first two blue loci, D3S1358 and vWA have amplified successfully but there is no FGA allele. This profile is from human muscle tissue that had been exposed to high temperatures and has degraded to the extent that there is very little or no DNA that is 200 bp or longer [30].

The interpretation of degraded profiles can be difficult and particular attention has to be taken when homozygous loci are detected – are they really homozygous and not heterozygous with one of the alleles having dropped out? When the levels are

Figure 7.13 The D18S51 locus dropped out when profiled using (a) the AmpFℓSTR® Identifiler®, but was successfully analysed using (b) the AmpFℓSTR® MiniFiler™

very low PCR amplification is carried out in duplicate or even triplicate to minimize the possibility of generating an incorrect profile.

To assist with the analysis of degraded DNA, a series of multiplexes have been developed with the primers positioned close to the core repeats of the STRs, thereby minimizing the lengths of the amplicons [31–35]. The combination of the standard STR multiplexes with the shortened amplicons can increase the amount of information recovered from a particular sample (Figure 7.13).

PCR inhibition

In addition to DNA degradation, if the DNA extraction procedure does not remove chemicals that interfere with the PCR, inhibition can result (Figure 7.14) (see Chapter 5). Inhibition can be difficult to differentiate from DNA degradation, although the use of real-time quantification can be used to detect inhibitors (see Chapter 4).

Figure 7.14 The same DNA extract was amplified in the presence of (a) 0 ng/µl humic acid; (b) 8 ng/µl humic acid; and (c) 12 ng/µl humic acid. The humic acid causes inhibition; at a concentration of 8 ng/µl the profile has a similar appearance to the degraded profile in Figure 7.10, with reduced peak heights at the larger loci; at a concentration of 12 ng/µl the profile is almost completely absent

References

1. Shinde, D. Lai YL, Sun FZ, Arnheim N. (2003) Taq DNA polymerase slippage mutation rates measured by PCR and quasi-likelihood analysis: (CA/GT)(n) and (A/T)(n) microsatellites. *Nucleic Acids Research*, **31**, 974–980.
2. Hauge, X.Y. and Litt, M. (1993) A Study of the origin of shadow bands seen when typing dinucleotide repeat polymorphisms by the PCR. *Human Molecular Genetics*, **2**, 411–415.
3. Schlotterer, C. and Tautz, D. (1992) Slippage synthesis of simple sequence DNA. *Nucleic Acids Research*, **20**, 211–215.
4. Applied Biosystems (1999) AmpFlSTR SGM Plus™ PCR Amplification Kit – User's Manual.
5. Gill, P., Sparkes, R. and Kimpton, C. (1997) Development of guidelines to designate alleles using an STR multiplex system. *Forensic Science International*, **89**, 185–197.

6. Bohnert, M., Faller-Marquardt, M., Lutz, S., Amberg, R., Weisser, H.J. and Pollak, S. (2001) Transfer of biological traces in cases of hanging and ligature strangulation. *Forensic Science International*, **116**, 107–115.

7. Esslinger, K.L., Siegel, J.A., Spillane, H. and Stallworth, S. (2004) Using STR analysis to detect human DNA from exploded pipe bomb devices. *Journal of Forensic Science*, **49**, 481–484.

8. van Oorschot, R.A.H. and Jones, M.K. (1997) DNA fingerprints from fingerprints. *Nature*, **387**, 767–767.

9. Wiegand, P. and Kleiber, M. (1997) DNA typing of epithelial cells after strangulation. *International Journal of Legal Medicine*, **110**, 181–183.

10. Gill, P. (2001) Application of low copy number DNA profiling. *Croatian Medical Journal*, **42**, 229–232.

11. Gill, P., Whitaker, J., Flaxman, C., Brown, N. and Buckleton, J. (2000) An investigation of the rigor of interpretation rules for STRs derived from less than 100 pg of DNA. *Forensic Science International*, **112**, 17–40.

12. Kloosterman, A.D. and Kersbergen, P. (2003) Efficacy and limits of genotyping low copy number DNA samples by multiplex PCR of STR loci. *International Congress Series*, **1239**, 795–798.

13. Whitaker, J.P., Cotton, E.A. and Gill, P. (2001) A comparison of the characteristics of profiles produced with the AmpFℓSTR (R) SGM Plus (TM) multiplex system for both standard and low copy number (LCN) STR DNA analysis. *Forensic Science International*, **123**, 215–223.

14. Gill, P., Brenner, C.H., Buckleton, J.S., Carracedo, A., Krawczak, M., Mayr, W.R. *et al.* (2006) DNA commission of the International Society of Forensic Genetics: recommendations on the interpretation of mixtures. *Forensic Science International*, **160**, 90–101.

15. Caddy, B., Taylor, G.R., Linacre, A.M.T. (2008) A review of the science of low template DNA analysis, (Office, H., ed).

16. Clayton, T.M., Whitaker, J.P., Sparkes, R. and Gill, P. (1998) Analysis and interpretation of mixed forensic stains using DNA STR profiling. *Forensic Science International*, **91**, 55–70.

17. Lygo, J.E., Johnson, P.E., Holdaway, D.J., Woodroffe, S., Whitaker, J.P., Clayton, T.M. *et al.* (1994) The validation of short tandem repeat (STR) loci for use in forensic casework. *International Journal of Legal Medicine*, **107**, 77–89.

18. Sparkes, R., Kimpton, C., Gilbard, S., Carne, P., Andersen, J., Oldroyd, N. *et al.* (1996) The validation of a 7-locus multiplex STR test for use in forensic casework. 2. Artefacts, casework studies and success rates. *International Journal of Legal Medicine*, **109**, 195–204.

19. Sparkes, R., Kimpton, C., Watson, S., Oldroyd, N., Clayton, T., Barnett, L. *et al.* (1996) The validation of a 7-locus multiplex STR test for use in forensic casework. 1. Mixtures, ageing, degradation and species studies. *International Journal of Legal Medicine*, **109**, 186–194.

20. Evett, I.W., Gill, P.D. and Lambert, J.A. (1998) Taking account of peak areas when interpreting mixed DNA profiles. *Journal of Forensic Science*, **43**, 62–69.

21. Gill, P., Sparkes, R., Pinchin, R., Clayton, T., Whitaker, J. and Buckleton, J. (1998) Interpreting simple STR mixtures using allele peak areas. *Forensic Science International*, **91**, 41–53.

22. Bill, M., Gill, P., Curran, J., Clayton, T., Pinchin, R., Healy, M. *et al.* (2005) PENDULUM – a guideline-based approach to the interpretation of STR mixtures. *Forensic Science International*, **148**, 181–189.

23. Clayton, T.M., Guest, J.L., Urquhart, A.J. and Gill, P.D. (2004) A genetic basis for anomalous band patterns encountered during DNA STR profiling. *Journal of Forensic Science*, **49**, 1207–1214.

24. Huel, R.L.M., Basic, L., Madacki-Todorovic, K., Smajlovic, L., Eminovic, I., Berbic, I. *et al.* (2007) Variant alleles, triallelic patterns, and point mutations observed in nuclear short tandem repeat typing of populations in Bosnia and Serbia. *Croatian Medical Journal*, **48**, 494–502.

25. Rolf, B., Wiegand, P. and Brinkmann, B. (2002) Somatic mutations at STR loci – a reason for three-allele pattern and mosaicism. *Forensic Science International*, **126**, 200–202.

26. Zamir, A., Shpitzen, M., Oz, C., Motro, U., Meiner, V. and Gafny, R. (2002) Presentation of a three-banded allele pattern – Analysis and interpretation. *Journal of Forensic Science*, **47**, 824–826.

27. Castella, V., Lesta, MdM and Mangin, P. (2009) One person with two DNA profiles: a(nother) case of mosaicism or chimerism. *International Journal of Legal Medicine*, **123**, 427–430.

28. Rubocki, R.J., McCue, B.J., Duffy, K.J., Shepard, K.L., Shepherd, S.J. and Wisecarver, J.L. (2001) Natural DNA mixtures generated in fraternal twins in utero. *Journal of Forensic Science*, **46**, 120–125.

29. Goodwin, W., McFarlane, J. and Roberts, J. (2003) The identification of a US serviceman recovered from the Holy Loch, Scotland. *Science and Justice*, **43**, 45–47.

30. Goodwin, W., Linacre, A. and Vanezis, P. (1999) The use of mitochondrial DNA and short tandem repeat typing in the identification of air crash victims. *Electrophoresis*, **20**, 1707–1711.

31. Butler, J.M., Shen, Y. and McCord, B.R. (2003) The development of reduced size STR amplicons as tools for analysis of degraded DNA. *Journal of Forensic Science*, **48**, 1054–1064.

32. Coble, M.D. and Butler, J.M. (2005) Characterization of new MiniSTR loci to aid analysis of degraded DNA. *Journal of Forensic Science*, **50**, 43–53.

33. Dixon, L.A., Dobbins, A.E., Pulker, H.K., Butler, J.M., Vallone, P.M. and Coble, M.D. (2006) Analysis of artificially degraded DNA using STRs and SNPs – results of a collaborative European (EDNAP) exercise. *Forensic Science International*, **164**, 33–44.

34. Drabek, J., Chung, D.T., Butler, J.M. and McCord, B.R. (2004) Concordance study between Miniplex assays and a commercial STR typing kit. *Journal of Forensic Science*, **49**, 859–860.

35. Gill, P., Fereday, L., Morling, N. and Schneider, P.M. (2006) The evolution of DNA databases – recommendations for new European STR loci. *Forensic Science International*, **156**, 242–244.

8 Statistical interpretation of STR profiles

Once it has been established that two DNA profiles are the same, the significance of the match has to be estimated. This requires some knowledge of population genetics and some statistical analysis of the data. This chapter will briefly cover the fundamental concepts involved with estimating the frequency of an STR profile in a given population.

Population genetics

It is necessary from the outset to define what is meant by a population. In the context of forensic genetics a population can be described as a group of people sharing common ancestry. In forensic terms the classification of a population within a country is usually quite broad, and many subgroups that can differ in language, culture and religion are placed together and classified as, for example Caucasian, sub-Saharan African and East Asian.

The Hardy–Weinberg law

Population genetics can be defined as the study of factors affecting the allele and genotype frequencies of different genetic loci in a population. The Hardy–Weinberg Law (HW law), also called the Hardy–Weinberg principle, provides a simple mathematical representation of the relationship of genotype and allele frequencies within an ideal population [1–3] and is central to forensic genetics. The HW law states that within a randomly mating population the genotype frequencies at any single genetic locus remain constant. When a population is obeying the HW law it is said to be in Hardy–Weinberg equilibrium (HWE). Importantly, when a population is in HWE, the genotype frequencies can be predicted from the allele frequencies. This relationship can be represented in a Punnett square (Figure 8.1).

The polymorphic STR loci used in forensic genetics have multiple alleles; however, the genotype frequency of a homozygote can be calculated using p^2 and that of

An Introduction to Forensic Genetics Second Edition   William Goodwin, Adrian Linacre and Sibte Hadi
© 2011 John Wiley & Sons, Ltd

	A ($p = 0.6$)	B ($q = 0.4$)
A ($p = 0.6$)	AA ($p^2 = 0.6^2 = 0.36$)	AB ($pq = 0.6 \times 0.4 = 0.24$)
B ($q = 0.4$)	AB ($pq = 0.6 \times 0.4 = 0.24$)	BB ($q^2 = 0.4^2 = 0.16$)

Figure 8.1 A Punnet square showing the relationship between alleles A and B, along with all the possible resulting genotypes. If allele A occurs at a frequency (p) of 0.6 and allele B occurs at frequency (q) of 0.4 then it is possible to estimate that the population will contain individuals with genotypes AA, AB and BB at frequencies of 0.36, 0.48 and 0.16 respectively. Each homozygote appears only once, hence p^2, or q^2. The heterozygote will be represented twice, hence $2pq$

heterozygotes can be calculated using $2pq$, removing the need to construct elaborate Punnet squares.

Deviation from the Hardy–Weinberg equilibrium

The HW law states that certain conditions must be met. These are:

- the population is infinitely large;
- random mating occurs within the population;
- the population is free from the effects of migration;
- there is no natural selection; and
- no mutations occur.

Clearly no human population will meet these criteria and all will deviate from the HW equilibrium to a greater or lesser extent.

Infinitely large population

A consequence of finite population size is that the frequency of alleles will change through a process known as random genetic drift, where the frequency of any given allele will increase or decrease through chance events. The effect of genetic drift is more pronounced in smaller populations [4]. However, most populations are sufficiently large for allele frequencies not to be significantly affected. Even in relatively small isolated human populations, it has been shown that alleles that are present at a frequency of more than 1% are rarely lost in recently diverged populations [5, 6].

Random mating

Humans clearly do not mate completely randomly. However, because STR genotypes do not have any impact on a person's phenotype, such as height, strength or intelligence, selection of an STR through sexual selection is unlikely and has not been demonstrated.

No migration

Human history is full of migrations and this obviously can lead to changes in the gene pools of populations. If two distinct populations are living in the same geographical area and they have different allele frequencies, each population can be in HWE. If the two different populations are not recognized within the larger population and are not treated as separate populations, deviation from the HWE may be apparent; this is known as the Wahlund effect [7–9]. If random admixture occurs between the two populations, the admixed population would be in HWE after one generation. In reality, where two populations have differences in language, culture or religion, admixture is normally a much longer process.

Natural selection

At some loci in the human genome the effect of selective pressures can be detected, for example lactase persistence that is present in populations where milk has been a sustained part of the diet [10, 11]. Mutations that can confer disease resistance can also exhibit strong selection effects. The mutation CCR5-Δ32, which is thought to offer protection against the haemorrhagic plague that led to vast numbers of Europeans dying between 1347 and 1670 AD, occurs at a frequency of almost zero in Asian, African and American Indian populations, whereas it is present at a frequency of 0.16 (16%) in European populations [12]. However, the loci that are used for forensic testing are not located within functionally important regions of the genome and there is no evidence that they are under selective pressure [13].

Mutation

Mutation at STR loci is relatively rapid and it is the instability at these loci that leads to their high levels of polymorphisms – a trait that makes them valuable genetic markers. However, the mutation rates of STRs are still relatively low at less than 0.2% per generation and do not have a significant effect on the allelic frequencies within a gene pool of different or even mixed populations [14–18].

Statistical tests to determine deviation from the Hardy–Weinberg equilibrium

Given that no human population can meet the requirements of the HW law can we then use it to calculate genotype proportions based on allele frequencies? The answer from most forensic scientists is yes – because we can empirically measure the predicted genotype frequencies under HWE and detect if there is a significant amount of deviation.

Many statistical tests have been developed to calculate the deviation of the allelic frequencies from HWE. These include the goodness-of-fit test (also called the chi square test), homozygosity test, likelihood ratio test and the exact test [19, 20]. However, when analysing polymorphic STR loci these tests do not have the required sensitivity because there are many undetected genotypes and numerous genotypes that are detected at very low frequencies at each locus. The multi-locus exact test was developed and can detect deviation from HWE when a large dataset is tested [21, 22]. Significant deviations from HWE have not been detected in the vast majority of populations, including some with high levels of consanguinity [23–25]. An exact test will not detect variations from HWE in small datasets, unless the deviation is extreme, and therefore conclusions from performing the exact test should not be over interpreted.

Estimating the frequencies of STR profiles

In forensic DNA analysis the HWE is used along with an allele frequency database to calculate genotype frequencies. An allelic frequency database is constructed by measuring the occurrence of alleles within the defined population. It has been recommended that a database of at least 200 alleles per locus (or 100 individuals) be used for a particular population when using the database for generating the statistical estimates of the strength of DNA evidence [26]. The larger the database, the more representative of the population it will be, and current practice dictates that several hundred individuals should be sampled when creating an allelic frequency database [27]. These people should not be direct relations; therefore siblings or mother and child, and so on combinations should not be incorporated into an allele frequency database.

Using the HWE, the expected genotype frequency at each locus is calculated using the observed allele frequencies. Using these frequencies along with the above HWE equations, we can calculate the frequency of a STR profile. If we take the profile that was analysed in Chapter 6, the genotype proportions for each locus are calculated using p^2 for the homozygote and $2pq$ for the heterozygote loci (Table 8.1). The overall profile frequency is calculated by multiplying the genotype frequency at each locus. This multiplication is termed the product rule; it is possible because the inheritance of alleles at each locus is independent of the other loci.

There have been some challenges to the approach presented above, namely that the inaccurate estimation of allelic frequencies can lead to inaccurate profile frequency estimates. To overcome this problem several methods have been employed that take into consideration the limitations in allele frequency estimates.

Corrections to allele frequency databases

Allelic frequencies are calculated by measuring a number of alleles in the target population. The more alleles that are measured as a part of the allelic frequency database the more accurate it will be. However, it is impracticable to measure all of

Table 8.1 The profile frequency is estimated using the principles of the Hardy–Weinberg law and an allele frequency database that was constructed using 400 alleles. Because the loci do not display any linkage and appear to be inherited independently of each other, the product rule can be used, multiplying each genotype frequency together to calculate the overall profile frequency

Locus	Allele	Allele frequency	HWE	Genotype frequency
D3S1358	15	0.2825	$2pq$	0.1257
	17	0.2225		
vWA	14	0.0850	$2pq$	0.0425
	17	0.2500		
D16S539	11	0.2975	$2pq$	0.1041
	13	0.1750		
D2S1338	24	0.1000	$2pq$	0.0240
	25	0.1200		
D8S1179	11	0.0625	$2pq$	0.0434
	13	0.3475		
D21S11	30	0.2625	$2pq$	0.0551
	31.2	0.1050		
D18S51	14	0.1675	$2pq$	0.0477
	15	0.1425		
D19S433	14	0.3275	$2pq$	0.0164
	15.2	0.0250		
TH01	9	0.1375	$2pq$	0.0963
	9.3	0.3500		
FGA	21	0.1775	p^2	0.0315
	21	0.1775		
		Profile frequency		7.579×10^{-14}

the alleles in a large population and the frequencies are only estimates, and prone to inaccuracies due to the limited size of the database. For common alleles the impact is small, but with rare alleles, which can easily be under-represented in a frequency database, the impact of limited sampling can have a large effect. It should be noted that the deficiencies in the frequency databases can also lead to over-representation of allele frequencies but, as a general principle, when we are estimating the significance of forensic evidence the emphasis is not to over-state the strength of the evidence. Different approaches have been taken to overcome the limitations of allele frequency databases. These include the allele frequency ceiling principle, the Balding size bias correction [28], allowing for the effects of subpopulations [29] and using a maximum profile frequency [30].

Allele ceiling principle

Very rare alleles may not appear at all in the frequency database. If a rare allele not previously represented on the frequency database is detected in a crime scene sample then the frequency of the allele would be zero – which cannot be the case! A mechanism must be put in place to deal with this situation. One approach is to set a minimal allele frequency. The minimum frequency values that are used vary from population to population but are typically around 0.01 (1%). Any allele occurring with a frequency of less than 0.01 will be adjusted to this figure. An alternative approach is to use a minimal allele count, for example five alleles being the smallest number of alleles that is considered: the allele frequency is simply calculated using the formula $5/2N$, where N is the number of individuals in the database [31].

Simple correction for sampling bias

Allele frequency databases are relatively small when compared with the populations from which they are drawn and therefore there remain sampling uncertainties. A simple method for addressing such uncertainties, which are inherent in allele frequency databases, is suggested by Balding [28]. The allelic information in the evidential material is incorporated into the database to adjust for the potential under-representation of alleles.

When there are matching DNA profiles there must be two DNA profiles: one from the crime scene and one from the reference sample. The alleles from these profiles are added to the allelic frequency database. By adding both profiles we are making the assumption that the material found at the crime scene did not come from the suspect. If we look at the profile in Table 8.1, at the vWA locus is a heterozygous locus with alleles 14 and 17; these have frequencies of 0.0850 and 0.2500, respectively. By multiplying the allele frequency with the total number of alleles in the database, we can calculate that the numbers of observed alleles in the database are 34/400 for allele 14 and 100/400 for allele 17. We now have two profiles to add to the database; we have seen a total of four new alleles: 14, 17 in the crime scene sample and also 14, 17 in the suspect's sample. These can be added to the database and the frequency recalculated. The database now has 36 observations of allele 14 out of a total of 404 observed alleles, which leads to an allele frequency of 0.090. Similarly, for allele 17 we now have 102/404, which gives us an allele frequency of 0.2525. This procedure is repeated for each heterozygous locus.

In Table 8.1 the FGA locus is homozygous, and in the original database we have 71/400 observations but now need to add four more observations (21, 21 and 21, 21) to both the frequency of allele 21 and the total number of alleles, so the new frequency is $75/404 = 0.1856$. The profile is recalculated using the correction method in Table 8.2.

The Balding correction for size bias has the greatest impact when the database is made from a small number of alleles or when the allele is rare. If the allele is common and the database is large, the effect is negligible.

The above methods both compensate for the limitations of allele frequency databases that are caused by sampling effects. Other more complex methods, such as calculating the 95% confidence interval, can be employed but are not widely used [31, 32].

Subpopulations

In addition to correcting for sampling effect, it may also be necessary to allow for the presence of subpopulations when calculating profile frequencies. Even within

Table 8.2 The profile frequency has been recalculated from Table 8.1 using the Balding correction for sampling bias. The impact of this correction factor is greatest on the rare alleles

Locus	Alleles	Allele frequency	Allele count	Corrected allele frequency	HWE	Genotype proportion
D3S1358	15	0.2825	113	115/404 = 0.2847	$2pq$	0.1282
	17	0.2225	89	91/404 = 0.2252		
vWA	14	0.0850	34	36/404 = 0.0891	$2pq$	0.0450
	17	0.2500	100	102/404 = 0.2525		
D16S539	11	0.2975	119	121/404 = 0.2995	$2pq$	0.1068
	13	0.1750	70	72/404 = 0.1782		
D2S1338	24	0.1000	40	42/404 = 0.1040	$2pq$	0.0257
	25	0.1200	48	50/404 = 0.1238		
D8S1179	11	0.0625	25	27/404 = 0.0668	$2pq$	0.0466
	13	0.3475	139	141/404 = 0.3490		
D21S11	30	0.2625	105	107/404 = 0.2649	$2pq$	0.0577
	31.2	0.1050	42	44/404 = 0.1089		
D18S51	14	0.1675	67	69/404 = 0.1708	$2pq$	0.0499
	15	0.1425	57	59/404 = 0.1460		
D19S433	14	0.3275	131	133/404 = 0.3292	$2pq$	0.0196
	15.2	0.0250	10	12/404 = 0.0297		
THO1	9	0.1375	55	57/404 = 0.1411	$2pq$	0.0992
	9.3	0.3500	140	142/404 = 0.3515		
FGA	21	0.1775	71	75/404 = 0.1856	p^2	0.0345
	21	0.1775	71	75/404 = 0.1856		
				Profile frequency		**1.4225×10^{-13}**

populations of the same broad ethnic group, the population is not homogeneous but comprises related subpopulations. The subpopulations form because people do not mate randomly but tend, for example, to have children with people from the same geographical area or same social group. Allelic databases are normally composed of samples that have been drawn from the general population, and not from one subpopulation, and therefore provide us with an average estimate of the allele frequencies in the whole population. The effect of subpopulations has been demonstrated as leading to errors in the estimation of profile frequencies [33]. In a subpopulation there is a higher degree of relatedness between individuals than there is to the whole population, that is a higher probability that two individuals would have some genetic markers in common through descent from a common ancestor (identical by descent) than by a random match (identical by state) [34]. To incorporate population substructure factor, and thereby account for variations in allele frequencies between different subpopulations, into the profile frequency calculations, a theta value (θ) is used to describe the degree of differentiation between subpopulations (the amount of inbreeding) [35, 36]. Actual levels of population substructure in human populations have been demonstrated to be low [31, 32, 37, 38]. A theta value of 0.01 is commonly used for seemingly homogeneous populations, whereas for more isolated/differentiated populations a theta value of 0.03 has been recommended [31]. It seems better to have empirical estimates of theta and use those for specific populations; however, that might not be practicable in all cases [39].

To calculate the profile frequencies that allow for subpopulations, the following equations are commonly used [21]:

For heterozygotes:

$$= \frac{2(\theta + (1 - \theta)p_A)(\theta + (1 - \theta)p_B)}{(1 + \theta)(1 + 2\theta)} \tag{8.1}$$

For homozygotes:

$$= \frac{(2\theta + (1 - \theta)p_A)(3\theta + (1 - \theta)p_A)}{(1 + \theta)(1 + 2\theta)} \tag{8.2}$$

We can use this to recalculate the profile frequency presented in Table 8.1: the calculations for the vWA and FGA locus are shown below with a theta value of 0.01.

vWA	FGA
$\dfrac{2(0.01 + (1 - 0.01)0.0850)(0.01 + (1 - 0.01)0.2500)}{(1 + 0.01)(1 + (2 \times 0.01))}$	$\dfrac{((2 \times 0.01) + (1 - 0.01)0.1775)((3 \times 0.01) + (1 - 0.01)0.1775)}{(1 + 0.01)(1 + (2 \times 0.01))}$
$\dfrac{2[0.0942][0.2575]}{(1.01)(1.02)}$	$\dfrac{2[0.0942][0.2575]}{(1.01)(1.02)}$
$\dfrac{0.0485}{1.0302} = 0.0471$	$\dfrac{0.0403}{1.0302} = 0.0391$

The impact of a theta value of 0.01 on this particular profile is a modest threefold increase in the profile frequency, whereas a theta value of 0.03 leads to a frequency that is over 20 times more common but still exceedingly rare (Table 8.3). It should be noted that the impact of applying theta to a profile frequency calculation differs between profiles (Figure 8.2). It should be noted that in a forensic context the theta term is often used interchangeably with the term F_{ST}.

The current practice in most legal systems is to use a theta value of between 0.01 and 0.03, apart from in exceptional circumstances where very high levels of

Table 8.3 The effect of different correction methods on the profile frequency calculated in Table 8.1. With this profile, applying a minimum allele frequency of 0.0125 would have no impact because the rarest allele frequency is 0.025

Calculation method	Profile frequency	Fold reduction relative to uncorrected frequency
Uncorrected	7.58×10^{-14}	–
Size bias	1.42×10^{-13}	2 (1.88)
Subpopulation: $\theta = 0.01$	2.44×10^{-13}	3 (3.29)
Subpopulation: $\theta = 0.03$	1.62×10^{-12}	21
Profile ceiling – 1 in 1 billion	1.00×10^{-9}	13 195

Figure 8.2 The SGM Plus frequencies from 252 UK Caucasians are shown with: ◆ no correction; ◆ theta (F_{ST}) 0.01; and ◆ theta (F_{ST}) 0.03. The impact of the theta correction varies – the greatest effect is with rare alleles and homozygous loci

inbreeding may have occurred. The impact of different theta (F_{ST}) values can be seen in Figure 8.2: as the theta increases the profile frequencies decrease.

Profile ceiling principle

In some countries, such as the UK, the approach has been to use a match probability of 1 in a billion (1 000 000 000). This approach is highly conservative [30]. It does have the advantage that individual profile frequencies do not have to be calculated because the value used is much lower than the most common profile frequency, even if conservative corrections are incorporated [32].

Which population frequency database should be used?

In some cases, the ethnic origins of material recovered from the crime scene are known: for example, if a woman has been sexually assaulted she can normally describe the assailant as white, black, Asian, and so on. In such a case, for example if the assailant was described as white, then it would be logical to use a white Caucasian allele frequency database to calculate the profile frequency. In other contexts, there may be no information about who could have left the material at the crime scene. In countries or regions having substantial populations with different ethnic backgrounds, a common practice is for the profile frequency to be calculated using an allele database for each major population group, and to use the most conservative profile frequency. If we take the example from Table 8.1, the allele frequency data used is from a white Caucasian database (USA); if we recalculate with allele frequency data representing an African American population we get a profile frequency of 3.36×10^{-16}, which is over 200 times less frequent than when we use the Caucasian frequency data. In this case it is clear that the Caucasian data provides a frequency estimate that is more conservative.

Conclusions

The methods that are employed for the correction of profile frequencies vary widely between different judicial systems and even different laboratories within the same judicial system. The allele ceiling principle, Balding correction, 95% confidence interval to correct for sampling error, accounting for population subdivision using theta, and the profile ceiling principle have all been used in forensic casework to calculate profile frequencies. For the profile that we have been using as an example in this chapter, the effect of the different correction methods can be seen in Table 8.3.

It should be noted that the impact of the different correction methods will vary depending on the individual profile and the size of the allele frequency database. The effect of the correction factors is to increase the frequency of the profile making it more common than it may actually be. The end result of analysing a profile is to produce a profile frequency, which is an estimate. Incorporating one or more of the correction factors into the profile frequency estimates reduces the chances of overstating the DNA evidence.

Further reading

Balding, D.J. (2005) *Weight-of-Evidence for Forensic DNA Profiles*, John Wiley & Sons, Ltd, Chichester, pp. 56–81.

Buckleton, J., Triggs, C.M. and Walsh, S.J. (2005) *Forensic DNA Evidence Interpretation*, CRC Press, pp. 341–347.

References

1. Hardy, G. (1908) Mendelian proportions in a mixed population. *Science*, **28**, 49–50.
2. Stern, C. (1943) The Hardy–Weinberg law. *Science*, **1997**, 137–138.
3. Weinberg, W. (1908) On the demonstration of heredity in man, in *(1963) Papers on Human Genetics* (ed. S.H. Boyer), Prentice Hall, pp. 4–15.
4. Helgason, A., Nicholson, G., Stefansson, K. and Donnelly, P. (2003) A reassessment of genetic diversity in Icelanders: Strong evidence from multiple loci for relative homogeneity caused by genetic drift. *Annals of Human Genetics*, **67**, 281–297.
5. Destro-Bisol, G., Boschi, I., Caglia, A., Tofanelli, S., Pascali, V. and Paoli, G. (2000) Microsatellite variation in Central Africa: an analysis of intrapopulational and interpopulational genetic diversity. *American Journal of Physical Anthropology*, **112**, 319–337.
6. Pardo, L.M., MacKay, I., Oostra, B., van Duijn, C.M. and Aulchenko, Y.S. (2005) The effect of genetic drift in a young genetically isolated population. *Annals of Human Genetics*, **69**, 288–295.
7. Chakraborty, R. (1987) Biochemical heterozygosity and phenotypic variability of polygenic traits. *Heredity*, **59**, 19–28.

8. Sinnock, P. (1975) Wahlund effect for 2-Locus model. *American Naturalist*, **109**, 565–570.

9. Smouse, P.E., Neel, J.V. and Liu, W. (1983) Multiple-locus departures from panmictic equilibrium within and between village gene pools of Amerindian tribes at different stages of agglomeration. *Genetics*, **104**, 133–153.

10. Tishkoff, S.A., Reed, F.A., Ranciaro, A., Voight, B.F., Babbitt, C.C., Silverman, J.S. *et al.* (2007) Convergent adaptation of human lactase persistence in Africa and Europe. *Nature Genetics*, **39**, 31–40.

11. Wooding, S.P. (2007) Following the herd. *Nature Genetics*, **39**, 7–8.

12. Duncan, S.R., Scott, S. and Duncan, C.J. (2005) Reappraisal of the historical selective pressures for the CCR5-Delta 32 mutation. *Journal of Medical Genetics*, **42**, 205–208.

13. Lohmueller, K.E. (2009) Graydon *et al.* provide no new evidence that forensic STR loci are functional. *Forensic Science International: Genetics*, **4**, 273–274.

14. Brinkmann, B., Klintschar, M., Neuhuber, F., Huhne, J. and Rolf, B. (1998) Mutation rate in human microsatellites: influence of the structure and length of the tandem repeat. *American Journal of Human Genetics*, **62**, 1408–1415.

15. Dauber, E.M., Bar, W., Klintschar, M., Neuhuber, F., Parson, W., Glock, B. *et al.* (2003) Mutation rates at 23 different short tandem repeat loci. *Progress in Forensic Genetics*, **9**, 565–567.

16. de Andrade, E.S., Gomes, A.V., Raposo, G., Mauricio-da-Silva, L., Silva, RdS (2009) Mutation rates at 14 STR loci in the population from Pernambuco, Northeast Brazil. *Forensic Science International: Genetics*, **3**, e141–e143.

17. Whittle, M.R., Romano, N.L. and Negreiros, V.A.C. (2004) Updated Brazilian genetic data, together with mutation rates, on 19 STR loci, including D10S1237. *Forensic Science International*, **139**, 207–210.

18. Yan, J.W., Liu, Y.C., Tang, H., Zhang, Q.X., Huo, Z.Y. and Hu, S.N. (2006) Mutations at 17 STR loci in Chinese population. *Forensic Science International*, **162**, 53–54.

19. Emigh, T.H. (1980) A comparison of tests for Hardy-Weinberg equilibrium. *Biometrics*, **36**, 627–642.

20. Wittke-Thompson, J.K., Pluzhnikov, A. and Cox, N.J. (2005) Rational inferences about departures from Hardy-Weinberg equilibrium. *American Journal of Human Genetics*, **76**, 967–986.

21. Guo, S.W. and Thompson, E.A. (1992) Performing the exact test of Hardy-Weinberg proportion for multiple alleles. *Biometrics*, **48**, 361–372.

22. Wigginton, J.E., Cutler, D.J. and Abecasis, G.R. (2005) A note on exact tests of Hardy-Weinberg equilibrium. *American Journal of Human Genetics*, **76**, 887–893.

23. Al-Obaidli, A., Sabbagh, A., Pravin, S. and Krishnamoorthy, R. (2009) Present day inbreeding does not forbid the forensic utility of commonly explored STR loci: a case study of native Qataris. *Forensic Science International: Genetics*, **4**, E11–E13.

24. Bindu, G.H., Trivedi, R. and Kashyap, V.K. (2007) Allele frequency distribution based on 17 STR markers in three major Dravidian linguistic populations of Andhra Pradesh, India. *Forensic Science International*, **170**, 76–85.

25. Haliti, N., Carapina, M., Masic, M., Strinovic, D., Klaric, I.M. and Kubat, M. (2009) Evaluation of population variation at 17 autosomal STR and 16 Y-STR haplotype loci in Croatians. *Forensic Science International: Genetics*, **3**, e137–e138.

26. Brinkmann, B. (1998) Overview of PCR-based systems in identity testing, *Forensic DNA Profiling Protocols*, Humana Press, pp. 105–120.

27. Schneider, P.M. (2007) Scientific standards for studies in forensic genetics. *Forensic Science International*, **165**, 238–243.

28. Balding, D.J. (1995) Estimating products in forensic identification using DNA profiles. *Journal of the American Statistical Association*, **90**, 839–844.

29. Balding, D.J. and Nichols, R.A. (1994) DNA profile match probability calculation - how to allow for population stratification, relatedness, database selection and single bands. *Forensic Science International*, **64**, 125–140.

30. Foreman, L.A. and Evett, I.W. (2001) Statistical analysis to support forensic interpretation for a new ten-locus STR profiling system. *International Journal of Legal Medicine*, **114**, 147–155.

31. National Research Council (1996) *The Evaluation of Forensic DNA Evidence*, National Academy Press.

32. Gill, P., Foreman, L., Buckleton, J.S., Triggs, C.M. and Allen, H. (2003) A comparison of adjustment methods to test the robustness of an STR DNA database comprised of 24 European populations. *Forensic Science International*, **131**, 184–196.

33. Curran, J.M., Buckleton, J.S. and Triggs, C.M. (2003) What is the magnitude of the subpopulation effect? *Forensic Science International*, **135**, 1–8.

34. Triggs, C.M. and Buckleton, J.S. (2002) Logical implications of applying the principles of population genetics to the interpretation of DNA profiling evidence. *Forensic Science International*, **128**, 108–114.

35. Buckleton, J.S., Curran, J.A. and Walsh, S.J. (2006) How reliable is the sub-population model in DNA testimony? *Forensic Science International*, **157**, 144–148.

36. Tvedebrink, T. (2009) Overdispersion in allelic counts and θ-correction in forensic genetics. *Forensic Science International: Genetics Supplement Series*, **2**, 455–457.

37. Foreman, L.A. and Lambert, J.A. (2000) Genetic differentiation within and between four UK ethnic groups. *Forensic Science International*, **114**, 7–20.

38. Foreman, L.A., Lambert, J.A. and Evett, I.W. (1998) Regional genetic variation in Caucasians. *Forensic Science International*, **95**, 27–37.

39. Zhivotovsky, L.A., Malyarchuk, B.A., Derenko, M.V., Wozniak, M. and Grzybowski, T. (2009) Developing STR databases on structured populations: the native South Siberian population versus the Russian population. *Forensic Science International: Genetics*, **3**, e111–e116.

9 Evaluation and presentation of DNA evidence

The final stage in any criminal case is the presentation of the evidence to the court. The way in which DNA evidence is presented has been, and still can be, a contentious subject. The evaluation process and the wording of the court reports and statements will be affected by both the judicial system and the prevailing approach to DNA evidence; this varies considerably between different countries. This chapter is designed as an introduction to the field and will guide the reader through the basics of the evaluation of DNA evidence.

Hierarchies of propositions

Any statement on the strength of the DNA evidence must be considered in the context of the case. DNA evidence should not be considered in isolation as it is affected by many factors such as the type of biological material, method and time of deposition and the substrate on which it was deposited.

There are three hierarchies of propositions in relation to biological material that can be considered in a criminal trial [1, 2]:

(1) **Source level**: from which individual did the biological material originate?

(2) **Activity level**: what activity led to the deposition of the biological material?

(3) **Offence level**: did the suspect commit the offence?

The hierarchies can be applied when, for example, considering a bloodstain found on the clothing of a suspect alleged to have committed an assault. The DNA evidence may assist in determining the most likely source of the stain. The size, shape and position of the stain may assist with determining the activity associated with the stain, that is how was it transferred and does this support an allegation of kicking or punching. The third hierarchical statement is that of offence: did the suspect commit the offence? The first hierarchical level can be addressed by DNA analysis and in many cases the second hierarchical level can be addressed to some extent by the

An Introduction to Forensic Genetics Second Edition   William Goodwin, Adrian Linacre and Sibte Hadi
© 2011 John Wiley & Sons, Ltd

forensic scientist, for example by the interpretation of blood spatter patterns, but the third level is the provenance of the court and at no time should an expert witness comment whether the defendant is guilty of the offence. This is clearly the task of the court to consider [3, 4].

To answer the first question, there are currently three approaches to the evaluation of DNA evidence. The three approaches are termed:

- the frequentist approach;

- the likelihood approach; and

- the Bayesian approach.

The frequentist approach

The profile frequency is presented as a random match probability, which can be taken as the reciprocal of the profile frequency.

$$\text{Random match probability} = \frac{1}{profile\ frequency} \tag{9.1}$$

Before the advent of DNA profiling, the results of blood groups and protein polymorphisms were expressed as random match probabilities; so, for example, a report might state that 'approximately 1 in 250 unrelated people will share this blood type'. It was natural to use this same wording with the advent of DNA analysis. In simple terms the frequentist approach describes the chance of a coincidental random match. Random match probability (also called random occurrence ratio) is the probability of a person, selected at random, having the same profile as the defendant [5].

If we take a profile with a frequency of 0.000 001 the random match probability will be:

$$\text{Random match probability} = \frac{1}{0.000001} = 1 \text{ in } 1\,000\,000$$

The use of multiplex STR kits can lead to match probabilities of hundreds of billions – far larger numbers than there are people on the planet.

If we take the profile from Chapter 8, after correction for subpopulation effects ($\theta = 0.01$) the random match probability will be:

$$\text{Random match probability} = \frac{1}{0.000000000000244} = 1 \text{ in } 4\,098\,360\,656\,000$$

In the UK the approach to such large numbers has been to employ a ceiling principle so that a figure of 1 in 1 billion is always quoted when describing a match based on a full SGM Plus® profile. There is little scientific merit to this approach but it is considered pragmatic. An example of a statement that is used in criminal reports in the UK is presented in the match probability statement.

Match probability statement

DNA analysis of the bloodstain from the crime scene gave a full DNA profile that matched that of the suspect. If this blood did not come from the suspect then the STR profile must match by chance. It is estimated that the chance of obtaining these matching profiles if the blood came from a random person unrelated to the suspect is in the order of 1 in 1 billion (a billion is a thousand million).

The frequentist approach has the advantage that when dealing with small numbers the phraseology can be understood. It should be noted that part of the duty of the forensic scientist is to make the strength of the evidence understood by the jury or a judge and, therefore, to that extent the frequency approach succeeds. Thus, quoting a random match probability figure of 1 in 1 million, for instance, is relatively simple for the jury to understand and picture. There are however a number of disadvantages with the approach. Take the example above, where the random match probability is 1 in 4 trillion. This leads to the observation that there are not 4 trillion people in the UK so what population is being described? Indeed there are only around 6.5 billion people on the planet at present.

Source attribution

One approach to the extremely strong evidence is once it reaches a defined point the prosecution can state that the bloodstain originated from a particular individual, that is they can attribute, with reasonable scientific certainty, the source of the forensic evidence to a given individual. Budowle *et al.* [6] provided some estimates for the profile frequencies that would be necessary – so, for example, a profile frequency of 3.9×10^{-11} or less would be unique in the 260 million individuals of the USA (with 99% confidence) [6]. In England, with a population of 50 million the target profile frequency for 99% confidence would be 2.0×10^{-10} or less [6]; all SGM® Plus® profiles shown in Figure 8.1 would meet this target.

However, current methods for determining source attribution have been criticized for not being sufficiently robust [7] and despite the advantages that source attribution may have, namely that it removes the need for a court to understand the meaning of extremely high random match probabilities, it has not gained widespread use.

Likelihood ratios

A likelihood ratio is the ratio of two competing hypotheses. In terms of a criminal case, it is the ratio of the prosecution hypothesis (H_p) and the defence hypothesis (H_d). The likelihood approach is a more logical way to interpret and present the profile frequency information as it considers an alternative scenario.

The three logical principles for the interpretation of DNA evidence and its quantification that have been suggested [8] are as follows:

(1) when evaluating DNA evidence two assumptions should be considered;

(2) the probability of occurrence of the evidence under each of the two assumptions should be quantified; and

(3) the ratio of the probabilities under two assumptions should be quantified and considered.

By considering the two propositions where one is the alternative of the other (the prosecution proposition compared with the defence proposition), then the probability of the evidence if the prosecution case is true can be determined. If the DNA profile of a crime scene sample matches a suspect's DNA profile then there can be two explanations.

(1) **Prosecution hypothesis (H_p)**: the DNA profile originated from the suspect.

(2) **Defence hypothesis (H_d)**: the DNA profile did not originate from the defendant but originated from another person.

The likelihood ratio is described in Equation 9.2. It is the probability (Pr) of the DNA evidence (E) given the hypothesis put forward by either the prosecution (H_p) or the defence (H_d):

$$\frac{\Pr(E|H_p)}{\Pr(E|H_d)} \tag{9.2}$$

The prosecution hypothesis is that the defendant left the biological material at the crime scene. The DNA profiles of the defendant and the evidence from the crime scene match, and therefore it is certain under the prosecution's hypothesis that the defendant left the material, hence $\Pr(E|H_p) = 1$. The probability of occurrence under the defence hypothesis is equal to the probability of observing the profile if its source was somebody other than the suspect in the population to which the defendant belongs. The ratio of the two probabilities is given by:

$$\text{Likelihood Ratio} = \frac{1}{profile\ frequency} \tag{9.3}$$

Let us assume that a certain crime scene stain yielded a DNA profile that has matched that of a suspect who is being prosecuted. The frequency of the matching DNA profile was 1 in a million. The likelihood ratio in this case would be:

$$\text{Likelihood Ratio} = \frac{1}{0.000001} = 1\,000\,000$$

Because with DNA evidence the probability under the prosecution's hypothesis is equal to 1, the value is the same as when calculating a random match probability; therefore, if we use the example from Chapter 8 we would have a likelihood ratio of over 4 trillion. The way that the value is expressed differs from a random match probability. The likelihood ratio would normally be expressed in a report with a statement, for example as in the likelihood ratio statement; the following statement is based on a likelihood ratio of 1 billion.

Likelihood ratio statement

DNA analysis of the bloodstain from the crime scene gave a full DNA profile that matched that of the suspect. If this blood did not come from the suspect then the STR profile must match by chance. The results of the DNA analysis are approximately 1 billion times more likely if the DNA came from the suspect than if the DNA came from a random unrelated male in the population (a billion is a thousand million).

The figure being quoted in a likelihood ratio is the odds in favour of the proposition put forward by the prosecution. When the statement reads that 'it is 1 million times more likely that the DNA came from the accused than if it came from any unrelated male', the figure of 1 million is not a probability but is an odds value, that is how many times more likely it is that the DNA matched the crime scene stain if it originates from the suspect, compared to coming from any other unrelated male. The frequency approach has a problem when the chance of a match, or the match probability, exceeds the total sample size. This is not the case when quoting odds in favour, as odds can reach near infinity. In a horse race with only five horses, one horse may have odds against of 10 to 1 and here the odds outweigh the number of possibilities.

The disadvantage with this statement is that it can seem to be cumbersome when presented to a jury. It is easy to make an error and state the probability that the evidential material came from the suspect instead of the probability that the DNA profile obtained from the evidential material matches that of the suspect.

Using the current multiplex STR kits that analyse between 10 and 15 STR loci, the match probabilities and therefore likelihood ratios are extremely high. In order to avoid some of these complications in presenting huge numbers, and also because it is easier for the scientist to express verbally the weight of the evidence, it has been suggested [3, 8] that verbal scales might be used for likelihood ratios as presented in Table 9.1.

The use of verbal equivalents is itself a contentious issue because of its subjective nature and also because some believe that it is encroaching on the role of the jury.

Table 9.1 Verbal scales for likelihood ratios

Likelihood ratios	Verbal equivalent
1–10	Limited support for prosecution hypothesis
10–100	Moderate support for prosecution hypothesis
100–1000	Moderately strong support for prosecution hypothesis
1000–10 000	Strong support for the prosecution hypothesis
>10 000	Very strong support for prosecution hypothesis

Further, there is no rationale for the boundaries, for example to discriminate between a likelihood ratio of 99 and one of 101.

The Bayesian approach

The Bayesian approach is favoured by many forensic scientists but has not gained widespread usage in the presentation of DNA evidence. The approach builds upon the likelihood but allows non-scientific data to be introduced in the form of prior odds. The non-scientific data will update the likelihood ratio to produce the final odds either in favour of or against the proposition put forward by the prosecution or defence (Equation 9.4).

$$\frac{Pr\,H_p}{Pr\,H_d} x \frac{Pr(E|H_p)}{Pr(E|H_d)} = \frac{Pr(H_p|E)}{Pr(H_d|E)}$$

(or prior odds × likelihood ratio = posterior odds)   (9.4)

Consider the case against Dennis Adams (*R* v *Adams* [1996] Cr. App. R., Part 3) in the UK where he was accused of a rape that occurred in 1991. The trial was in 1994 when the DNA profiling methodology was based upon VNTR analysis that pre-dated STR typing. The DNA evidence put forward by the prosecution was that the DNA profile occurred in 1 in 200 million of the population. Adams pleaded not guilty; he had an alibi and was not identified at an identity parade. The defence expert produced numerical values for the crime being committed by a local man, for the possibility of not being identified at the parade and for the alibi. All these prior probabilities were multiplied to determine the prior probability. The defence argued that the evidence (genetic and non-genetic) indicated the innocence of the accused. At the trial the judge allowed this to happen and directed the jury that they could use the Bayesian figure if they wished. Adams was found guilty.

The use of Bayesian evaluation of DNA evidence in the UK legal system has not been accepted and has led to successful appeals against convictions, including the above example, when the Appeal Court took the view that the use of Bayesian statistics trespassed on areas exclusively and peculiarly those of the jury. The relationship between different pieces of evidence was for the jury to decide and the mathematical formula might be applied differently by a different set of jurors. Jurors should evaluate the evidence by the joint application of their common sense and knowledge of the world to the material before them. A significant ruling was laid down in the English Courts following another appeal (*R v Doheny and Adams* [1996] EWCA Crim 728). A number of the relevant points can be summarized:

(1) The scientist should give the frequency of the occurrence with which the DNA profile is likely to be found in the population.

(2) It might be appropriate, if the scientist has the necessary data and statistical expertise, to say how many people might be found to have matching profiles in the United Kingdom or in a limited subgroup of individuals (the idea is to give the jury an estimate of how many people in the relevant section of the population are expected to have a matching profile and, therefore, could be the source of the stain).

(3) The jury would then decide, on all the information available, whether the stain originated from the suspect or some other individual with a matching profile.

(4) To help the jury, the judge might direct them along the following lines:

... if you accept the evidence that indicates there are only four or five (or whatever figure) men in the UK population from whom the stain could have originated and the suspect is one of them, are you sure the suspect left the stain or is it possible it was one of the other individuals in the small group who has a matching profile.

Two fallacies

When presenting evidence two errors can be committed if precise wording is not used; care should be taken to avoid committing the prosecutor's or defendant's fallacy.

Prosecutor's fallacy

This fallacy in describing the strength of the evidence is also called 'transposed conditional' [9]. If a horse is described as a four-legged animal it does not transpose that every four-legged animal is a horse. Similarly the statement 'the probability of gaining this DNA profile *if* it came from someone other than the suspect is 1 in 1 million', does not mean that 'the probability that the evidence came from someone other than the suspect is 1 in 1 million'. The first statement considers the probability of the evidence given the hypothesis and is correct, but the second statement considers the probability of the hypothesis given the evidence, and is a clear case of the prosecutor's fallacy.

In the case of Andrew Deen (*R v Deen* [1994] *The Times*, 10 January 1994) in the UK, the DNA analyst incorrectly defined match probability as the 'probability of the semen having originated from someone other than Andrew Deen'. In the examination in chief, the DNA analyst said 'the likelihood of (the source of the semen) being any other man but Andrew Deen is one in three million'. It is clear that the analyst transposed the condition of the hypothesis and it was one of the reasons that the conviction was quashed by the Court of Appeal.

As another example, consider the following dialogue from *R v Doheny and Adams* (*R v Doheny and Adams* [1996] EWCA Crim 728):

Q. Is it possible that the semen could have come from a different person from the person who provided the blood samples?

A. It is possible but it is so unlikely as to really not be credible. I can calculate; I can estimate the chances of this semen having come from a man other than the provider of the blood sample. I can work out the chances as being less than 1 in 27 million.

Instead of estimating the probability of semen (crime scene sample) matching blood (of the suspect) if the suspect was innocent, the DNA analyst was estimating the probability of the semen matching the suspect's blood if the suspect left the semen stain. For the population of the UK a match probability of 1 in 27 million means that other persons could have a matching profile and without other supporting evidence may not in itself provide sufficient evidence against the defendant. This however is a matter for the court to address and not the scientist. The prosecution expert witness thus inadvertently enhanced and misrepresented the probative value of the evidence [9]. It is therefore imperative that in order to avoid the prosecutor's fallacy, the scientists write their report carefully, and while answering any questions in the court keep their match probability or likelihood statements conditioned on 'if the defendant was innocent'.

Defendant's fallacy

If the match probability for a DNA profile was 1 in 27 million as it was in the case against Doheny, the defence could argue, for example, that three people in the UK might match the crime scene profile, the probability of the defendant being the donor of the crime scene sample is therefore only one-third, which is insufficient for proof beyond reasonable doubt. The issue with this statement is that nothing is known of these three people; whether they exist, where they live, what age they are, what sex they are and what opportunity they might have to leave their DNA at the scene.

Comparison of three approaches

The high statistical values that are attached to DNA profiles might seem intimidating and can unduly enhance the probative value of DNA evidence. This had led to heated debate over the way in which the evidence should be presented to a court.

The frequentist approach is straightforward and understandable by both a jury and a judge. For the reporting officer it is straightforward to state in court, and the opportunity for transposing the conditional and stating the prosecutor's fallacy is less than with the other two approaches. A disadvantage of the approach is that it does not consider two propositions where one is the alternative of the other. The likelihood ratio is a logical approach; it considers an alternative hypothesis. The Bayesian approach is the most logical way to incorporate all evidence in a case; it considers alternative hypotheses but it is difficult to calculate and conceptualize.

Further reading

Balding, D.J. (2005) *Weight-of-evidence for Forensic DNA Profiles*, John Wiley & Sons, Ltd, Chichester, pp. 145–156.

Buckelton, J., Triggs, C.M. and Walsh, S.J. (2005) *Forensic DNA Evidence Interpretation*, CRC Press, pp. 27–63.

References

1. Cook, R., Evett, I.W., Jackson, G., Jones, P.J. and Lambert, J.A. (1998) A model for case assessment and interpretation. *Science and Justice*, **38**, 151–156.
2. Evett, I.W., Jackson, G. and Lambert, J.A. (2000) More on the hierarchy of propositions: exploring the distinction between explanations and propositions. *Science and Justice*, **40**, 3–10.
3. Evett, I.W., Jackson, G., Lambert, L.A. and McCrossan, S. (2000) The impact of the principles of evidence interpretation on the structure and content of statements. *Science and Justice*, **40**, 233–239.
4. Taroni, F. and Aitken, C.G.G. (2000) DNA evidence, probabilistic evaluation and collaborative tests. *Forensic Science International*, **108**, 121–143.
5. Meester, R. and Sjerps, M. (2004) Why the effect of prior odds should accompany the likelihood ratio when reporting DNA evidence. *Law Probability and Risk*, **3**, 51–62.
6. Budowle, B., Chakraborty, R., Carmody, G. and Monson, K.L. (2000) Source attribution of a forensic DNA profile. *Forensic Science Communications*, **3**. http://www.fbi.gov/hq/lab/fsc/backissu/july2000/source.htm (accessed July 2010).
7. Triggs, C.M. and Buckleton, J.S. (2002) Logical implications of applying the principles of population genetics to the interpretation of DNA profiling evidence. *Forensic Science International*, **128**, 108–114.
8. Evett, I.W. and Weir, B.S. (1998) *Interpreting DNA Evidence – Statistical Genetics for Forensic Scientists*, Sinauer Associates, pp. 217–246.
9. Balding, D.J. and Donnelly, P. (1994) The prosecutor's fallacy and DNA evidence. *Criminal Law Review*, **1994**, 711–721.

10 Databases of DNA profiles

Several countries have developed national DNA databases that contain large numbers of DNA profiles: the UK and the USA national DNA databases, as of mid-2010, both contain the DNA profiles of over 5 million individuals. DNA databases that store STR profiles have emerged as a powerful tool in the investigation of crime. The effective use of the DNA database, in particular in the UK, has acted as a catalyst for the establishment and expansion of DNA databases in other countries. Currently there are DNA databases operating in almost every European country, the USA, Canada, Australia, South Africa and New Zealand. The Interpol DNA survey in 2008 found that 120 countries were using DNA typing of one form or another in criminal investigations, and 54 now operate a DNA database [1]. The range and types of samples collected varies from jurisdiction to jurisdiction as does the retention and use of the data. This chapter will examine the development and application of the UK National DNA Database (NDNAD), which is the first and most extensive database of its kind. It will briefly examine the development of databases worldwide.

The UK National DNA Database

The UK NDNAD was established in 1995 [2], shortly after STR profiling using six STR loci (the SGM) was introduced into criminal casework.

Rationale for criminal databases in the UK

There are several justifications for the time, effort and money that a criminal DNA database consumes.

- Criminals tend to reoffend – 90% of rapists have had a previous conviction; 50% of armed robbers have a previous conviction.

- The severity of crimes often increases – in many instances criminal activity starts at a young age with many criminals committing their first offence between 16 and 19 years of age.

An Introduction to Forensic Genetics Second Edition   William Goodwin, Adrian Linacre and Sibte Hadi
© 2011 John Wiley & Sons, Ltd

- A small number of criminals can be responsible for a large number of crimes – linking these crimes together can aid police investigations. This is particularly the case for burglaries, auto crimes and serious cases such as sexual assaults.

Legislation

The UK DNA database did not require specific statutes for its establishment, although the police service launched the national DNA database at the same time that the provisions of the Criminal Justice and Public Order Act 1994 came into force on 10 April 1995. Subsequent legislation has increased the scope of samples that may be collected and retained on the NDNAD.

Legislation in England and Wales[1]

1994 The Criminal Justice and Public Order Act
Within the UK the Police and Criminal Evidence (PACE) Act 1984, which governs the taking of samples from persons suspected of criminal activity, was amended so that a sample could be taken from anybody arrested for a recordable offence; previously samples were only taken if an individual was charged with a 'serious arrestable offence'. Significantly, it was also amended to reclassify saliva and mouth swabs as non-intimate, thus allowing the samples to be collected without consent and without the need for a medical practitioner.

1997 The Criminal Evidence (Amendment) Act
This allowed non-intimate samples to be collected from individuals currently in prison but convicted of an offence prior to the establishment of the NDNAD.

2001 Criminal Justice and Police Act
This allowed samples to be retained indefinitely, irrespective of whether the person was acquitted at trial, and from samples obtained from volunteers taking part in mass screens, provided that these volunteers gave their consent.

2003 Criminal Justice Act
Section 63 of the PACE Act (1984) was amended to allow the police to take a non-intimate sample from a person in police detention who has been arrested for, charged with, informed they will be reported for or convicted of a recordable offence. These powers came into force in 2004.

2005 Serious Organized Crime and Police Act
This made all offences arrestable; previously offences were categorized as non-arrestable, arrestable and serious arrestable. Also, extended legislation so

---

[1] Note: Some pieces of legislation only apply in England and Wales, with other parts of the UK differing in key aspects, such as retention policy.

that DNA profiles are retained on the database, even if the suspect has been cleared.

2009 European Court of Human Rights
In the appeal case of S and Marper, the European Court of Human Rights (ECHRs) ruled that the retention of samples collected from person for whom there was no criminal conviction was a violation of Article 8 and 14 of the Convention of Human Rights.

Criteria for entry onto the UK NDNAD

The original criterion for addition of a sample from an individual to the NDNAD was that the person had been arrested for an offence punishable by imprisonment. If the person was found not guilty at a subsequent trial, or the case was discontinued, then their profile would be removed. In 2001 the Criminal Justice and Police Act allowed samples to be retained on the NDNAD, even if the individual was not found guilty. The regulations were further relaxed in 2003 and 2005 with the Criminal Justice Act and Serious Organized Crime and Police Act. This led to an ever-increasing number of DNA profiles added to the NDNAD with a mix of those for whom there was a criminal conviction and those who provided a sample as part of an investigation but no further action was taken. As of 2010 the NDNAD contained the profiles of approximately 1 million individuals that had not been found guilty of any crime.

Challenges had been raised to the inclusion and retention policies of the NDNAD and in 2008 a landmark ruling was made by the ECHR in an appeal case by two individuals from England, S and Marper (S was under 10 years old when his samples were taken). The proposed response from the UK Home Office to the ECHR's ruling was that profiles of all those over 18 years convicted of a criminal offence to be retained indefinitely; all samples from those under 10 to be removed; profiles of those over 18 arrested but not convicted to be stored between 6 and 12 years; profiles from those between 10 and 18 stored either up to the eighteenth birthday or stored for 12 years, depending on the nature of the offence [3, 4].

In addition to the inclusion and retention policies of the NDNAD, ethical concerns have also been raised that the database discriminated against vulnerable sections of society – 75% of young black males between the ages of 15 and 34 are on the database, whereas only 22% of white males in the same age bracket are represented [5].

Technology underlying the NDNAD

The development of STR profiling was essential for the successful implementation of a large-scale DNA database. Attempts had been made to construct databases of VNTR profiles [6], and these did produce some matches. However, the difficulty of comparing VNTR profiles was a major limitation. STR profiles can be digitized very easily to create a digital code. This digital code allowed for the effective computerization of DNA profiles (see Chapter 6).

The UK NDNAD was established using the SGM multiplex, which analysed six STR loci and the amelogenin locus. The average match probability of SGM was 1 in 10^8 of the population, which for a population of 58 million within the UK was deemed acceptable. However, when six loci were used there were a number of coincidental (adventitious) matches.

Adventitious hits

In 1995 Raymond Easton was asked to donate a DNA profile as part of an investigation into a domestic dispute. Four years later a burglary at a home approximately 200 km from where Raymond Easton lived generated a DNA profile that was compared with the NDNAD. This profile matched that of Raymond Easton and he was accused of the crime. A match probability of 1 in 37 million was reported. At the time of the burglary, Raymond Easton was suffering from Parkinson's disease and was unable to walk more than 10 m unaided. This was an example of an adventitious hit. The test was conducted using the six SGM loci, but the chance that a similar adventitious cold hit will occur has been reduced greatly by extending the test to 10 loci [7].

In 1999, the six-locus SGM test was changed to the 10-locus SGM Plus® test. The chance that two DNA profiles from unrelated people will match at all 10 loci is less than 1 in 1 billion. To date no two people have been found to match at all 10 loci; however, matches to two or more people do occur if a partial DNA profile, recovered from poor-quality DNA, is searched against the NDNAD.

Operation of the NDNAD

The NDNAD has two main sets of data: profiles generated from evidence that has been collected from crime scenes (350 000 were retained in the database as of 31 March 2010) and profiles generated from individuals (4.85 million as of 31 March 2010 [8]).

A biological sample collected from a crime scene will be submitted for DNA analysis. The resulting DNA profile will be compared with those currently held on the NDNAD and if there is a match then this will be reported back to the police force that collected the sample (Figure 10.1).

Since 2000, on average the NDNAD has provided around 40 000 crime scene to individual matches each year (Figure 10.2). Although the intention had been to use the NDNAD to match samples from serious crimes such as sexual assaults and

Potential matches:

– Crime scene to suspect

– Crime scene to crime scene

– Suspect to suspect

Figure 10.1 Following entry onto the database the new samples are searched against all other samples on the NDNAD. Suspect to suspect matches will only occur when individuals have given incorrect details to the police about their identity unless a coincidental match occurs; to date no coincidental matches have been reported with a full SGM Plus® DNA profile

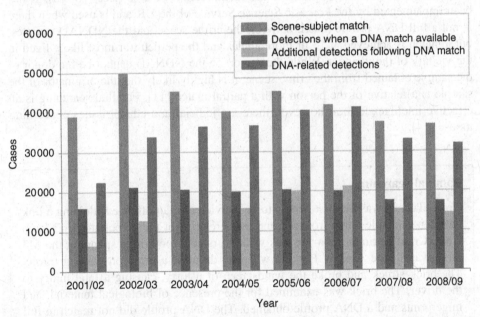

Figure 10.2 Number of cases are shown where a scene–subject match was recorded along with the cases that involved DNA evidence [8]; matches are not necessarily to a suspect and can be to people with a legitimate reason to be at the crime scene. Detections are shown where the crime was cleared up and a DNA match was available. Additional detections are achieved through the DNA link, for example when a suspect admits to further offences under questioning

murders, the addition of samples from high volume crime such as burglary resulted in an increase in DNA profiles on the NDNAD; the majority of matches are to high volume crime but there are invariably matches to more serious crimes such as murder, rape and assaults (Figure 10.3) [8, 9].

In the UK, approximately 1 in 20 people are on the NDNAD; given that over 80% of all samples on the NDNAD come from males and that there are approximately 30 million males in the total population, this equates to over 12% of the total male population [4, 8]. With such a large number of DNA profiles held on the NDNAD there is currently a 58% chance that a DNA profile obtained from an incident will match a DNA profile on the NDNAD.

Familial searching

Familial searching is based on the principle that family members share more of their DNA than more distantly related individuals and therefore searching a database using a close family member may enable the identification of a suspect [10–13]. It has been implemented by the Forensic Science Service of the UK and is used when there is not a full DNA profile match between the crime scene and the NDNAD samples, but a match is achieved at 15 or more alleles and the perpetrator most likely lived in the vicinity of the incident. While the person on the NDNAD cannot be the donor of the sample obtained from the crime scene, it is highly likely that the originator of the sample is a relative of the person with a partial match [11]. Familial searching is an effective intelligence tool; however, there are judicial and ethical issues concerning its use [14].

Familial searching

Craig Harman was the first person to be convicted of an offence following a link between a sample taken from a scene and a relative of the perpetrator. In March 2003, Craig Harman, then 19, was walking over a footbridge spanning the M3 motorway to the west of London when he dropped a brick on passing traffic. The brick struck and broke the windscreen of a lorry, causing a fatal injury to the driver. The brick was examined for the presence of biological material, and fingerprints and a DNA profile obtained. The DNA profile did not match in full with any person on the NDNAD but 16 of the 20 alleles matched a genetic relative of Craig Harman. A separate complete match was obtained between the samples obtained from the brick sample taken from Craig Harman after he was linked to the crime through the partial match. Craig Harman pleaded guilty to manslaughter.

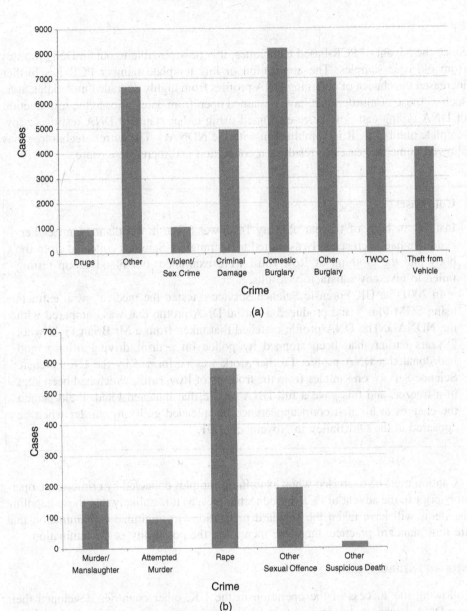

Figure 10.3 (a) The number of cases that were linked to one or more individuals through the NDNAD in 2007/2008 (TWOC: taken without owner's consent). (b) Shows a breakdown of the violent and sex crimes [8]

Cold cases

Since the advent of PCR-based techniques, it is now possible to obtain DNA profiles from old case samples. The application of low template number PCR has further increased the chance of obtaining DNA profiles from highly degraded material. Cases, such as those of murder, that have remained open from dates prior to the introduction of DNA typing can now be re-examined using either standard DNA testing or low template number PCR in combination with the NDNAD. The current technology has allowed numerous cases to result in a conviction and therefore closure.

Cold cases

In 1969 the body of 14-year-old Roy Tutill was found in woodland near Leatherhead. He had been sexually assaulted and strangled. Samples collected from the body and the clothing of Roy Tutill were examined, but blood group testing failed to give any satisfactory results.

In 2001 the UK Forensic Science Service retested the medical swab extracts using SGM Plus® and produced a partial DNA profile that was compared with the NDNAD. The DNA profile matched that taken from a Mr Brian Field who, 2 years earlier, had been stopped by police on a drink-driving offence and had donated a DNA profile. Further work was performed by the UK Forensic Science Service on samples from the trousers of Roy Tutill, which had been kept in a freezer, and this gave a full DNA profile that matched Field. Field denied the charges at his first court appearance but pleaded guilty to murder when he appeared at the Old Bailey in November 2001.

Caution must be exercised when examining samples collected by crime scene operators prior to the advent of PCR-based techniques, as it is unlikely that those handling the items will have taken the standard precautions to minimize contamination that are now standard practice, therefore increasing the possibility of contamination.

International situation

Following the success of the operation in the UK, other countries developed their own DNA databases. For many countries there was a need to enact special legislation leading to delays in the implementation of DNA databases [15].

US DNA database

The US Army established a database of their own in 1992 to identify missing persons in operation Desert Storm and this experience helped to pave the way for a national database within the USA. In 1994 the US congress passed the DNA Identification Act (Public Law 103 322), which enabled the establishment of CODIS. CODIS, which is the federally held DNA database, has expanded very quickly and comprises the National DNA Index System (NDIS), the State DNA Index System (SDIS) and the Local DNA Index System (LDIS). The information about each sample that is loaded onto the CODIS database includes a laboratory identifier, a specimen identifier, information to classify and review the integrity of the DNA record and the DNA profile itself. CODIS links local, state and federal crime laboratories. The FBI selected 13 STR loci (CODIS loci) for developing the database. Like the UK NDNAD there are two main segments called 'indices' of CODIS:

- The Forensic Index contains DNA profiles from crime scene samples.

- The Offender Index contains DNA profiles of individuals convicted of certain categories of violent crime, although now many States are expanding their databases and are profiling persons arrested for all felonies.

Other CODIS indices are:

- unidentified human remains;

- relatives of missing persons.

At the moment there are about 200 DNA laboratories around the USA that are designated and accredited as CODIS laboratories. These laboratories are validated according to the standards of FBI and are authorized to submit the DNA profile information into CODIS.

The situation in the USA as of July 2010 is:

- total number of offender profiles: 7 940 321

- total forensic profiles: 306 028.

When compared with the UK, the USA is a much larger jurisdiction and now contains more profiles. However, because of lack of funding, coherent structure and variable legal approaches, there have been lengthy delays in DNA profiling of casework samples that has led to massive backlogs. The president of the USA announced the 'President's DNA Initiative' in 2003 in order to enhance and streamline the use of DNA as a forensic tool and also signed an act to enhance the facilities for DNA databasing [16]. The main aims of this initiative were to clear the backlogs quickly and also to improve the capacity of the forensic laboratories for databasing the samples besides promoting research and development in the field; unfortunately, delays in processing samples have continued [17]. In spite of this, the number of samples has increased dramatically, and in terms of total samples on the database the USA has now by far the largest criminal database.

European databases

In mainland Europe, many countries have established DNA databases [18]. The Netherlands and Austria established their version of a DNA database in 1997, with Germany following 1 year later and Finland and Norway in 1999 [19]. Since the introduction of DNA databases in many European countries, the legislation governing the collection and retention of samples has also altered to facilitate the addition of samples onto the database and the circumstances in which the database can be searched: for example, in Germany, a judge is no longer required to sanction DNA typing of crime scene samples. Following the treaty of Prüm, there is increasing cooperation on sharing data between European countries.

Australian and New Zealand databases

New Zealand implemented a DNA database in 1996 along similar lines to that of the UK. The population is significantly smaller, but as a percentage of the population New Zealand is second only to the UK in terms of the number of DNA profiles held on its database. This is reflected in the fact that 63% of profiles loaded from crime scenes result in a match to an individual on the database. Australia was also rapid in developing DNA databases, although, in the first instance, as Australia is a federal country with six states and two territories, each state required to make an agreement with the other five states to allow the transmission of data between them, resulting in 49 separate pieces of legislation.

Cross-border databases

Criminals tend to operate in their own country but there are circumstances when crimes will be committed in more than one country. In order for criminal databases to be effective in these circumstances there is a need to share data. Interpol has been instrumental in facilitating cross-border comparisons of DNA profiles. The STR loci commonly used in the forensic community were combined to make the Interpol Standard Set of Loci (ISSOL); recommendations have been made to expand it from 7 to 10 loci [20]. In Europe the EU Council resolution 9192/01 calls upon European countries to use the European Standard Set (ESS), which are the same as the Interpol loci, as a minimum to enable international comparison of DNA profiles; the loci have been selected through the European Network of Forensic Science Institutes (ENFSIs) (Table 10.1).

The biggest obstacle to cross-border data sharing is now political rather than technical; developments like the treaty of Prüm have lead to increased sharing of data across borders and this is likely to continue.

Table 10.1 Core STR loci as defined by different agencies, which facilitate the sharing of DNA profiles across international borders. As databases increase in size there is a requirement for more loci to be added in order to avoid adventitious (false) matches

INTERPOL	ESS	ESS-extended	CODIS
D3S1358	D3S1358	D3S1358	D3S1358
TH01	TH01	TH01	TH01
D21S11	D21S11	D21S11	D21S11
D18S51	D18S51	D18S51	D18S51
vWA	vWA	vWA	vWA
D8S1179	D8S1179	D8S1179	D8S1179
FGA	FGA	FGA	FGA
–	–	D1S1656	–
–	–	D2S441	–
–	–	D10S1248	–
–	–	D12S391	–
–	–	D22S1045	–
–	–	–	TPOX
–	–	–	CSF1PO
–	–	–	D5S818
–	–	–	D7S820
–	–	–	D13S317
–	–	–	D19S433

Treaty of Prüm

The Treaty of Prüm was designed to allow the law enforcement agencies from the participating countries to have access to DNA, fingerprint and motor vehicle registration databases between the signature countries. The treaty signed in May 2005 by the Netherlands, Austria, Germany, Belgium, Luxembourg, Spain and France has since been joined by other member states: Finland, Italy, Portugal, Slovenia, Greece, Sweden, Bulgaria, Romania, Slovakia and Hungary have joined. The EU council has accepted to convert the information exchange part of the treaty into EU legislation. This leads ultimately to all 27 current members of the EU being party to this treaty.

The ESS of loci comprises seven loci with a commonality to those used currently (see Table 10.1). It is a requirement of the Treaty of Prüm that at least six of the seven loci must give a result. The increasing chance of adventitious hits due to the large cumulative DNA database in Europe has led to recommendations to type and exchange data for additional loci [21]. The drive towards sharing of data will further result in the standardization of the DNA loci used not only within one continent but worldwide.

Within 6 weeks of the Treaty of Prüm being operational Germany and Austria had exchanged data that led to 1500 DNA matches being reported, including 32 homicide cases and 23 rape/sexual assault cases [22].

Further reading

Williams, R. and Johnson, P. (2008) *Genetic Policing: The Use of DNA in Criminal Investigations*, Willan Publishing, London.

WWW resources

Interpol (DNA front page): http://www.interpol.int/Public/Forensic/DNA/
Federal Bureau of Investigation (CODIS Information): http://www.fbi.gov/hq/lab/codis/clickmap.htm
National Police Improvement Agency (National DNA Database (UK)): http://www.npia.police.uk/en/8934.htm
Association of Chief Police Officers of England, Wales and Northern Ireland: (National DNA Database report): http://www.acpo.police.uk/policies.asp
GeneWatch UK: http://www.genewatch.org

References

1. INTERPOL (2008) INTERPOL Global DNA Profiling Survey 2008 Key Facts (Public Version), INTERPOL, Lyon.
2. Werrett, D.J. (1997) The national DNA database. *Forensic Science International*, **88**, 33–42.
3. Information Commissioner's Office (2009) The Information Commissioner's Response to the Home Office Consultation Paper on the Retention, Use and Destruction of DNA Data and Fingerprints, Information Commissioner's Office, London.
4. Home Office (2009) Keeping the Right People on the DNA Database, Home Office, London.
5. Human Genetics Commission (2009) Nothing to Hide, Nothing to Fear? Department of Health, London.
6. Baechtel, F.S., Monson, K.L., Forsen, G.E., Budowle, B. and Kearney, J.J. (1991) Tracking the violent criminal offender through DNA typing profiles – a national database system concept, in *DNA Fingerprinting: Approaches and Applications* (eds T. Burke *et al.*), Birkhauser Verlag, pp. 356–360.
7. Staley, K. (2005) *The Police National DNA Database: Balancing Crime Detection, Human Rights and Privacy*, GeneWatch, Buxton.
8. National Policing Improvement Agency (2009) National DNA Database Annual Report 2007–2009.
9. Parliamentary Office of Science and Technology (2006) The National DNA Database, Parliamentary Office of Science and Technology, London.
10. Curran, J.M. and Buckleton, J.S. (2008) Effectiveness of familial searches. *Science and Justice*, **48**, 164–167.
11. Greely, H.T., Riordan, D.P., Garrison, N.A. and Mountain, J.L. (2006) Family ties: the use of DNA offender databases to catch offenders' kin. *Journal of Law Medicine and Ethics*, **34**, 248–262.
12. Reid, T.M., Baird, M.L., Reid, J.P., Lee, S.C. and Lee, R.F. (2008) Use of sibling pairs to determine the familial searching efficiency of forensic databases. *Forensic Science International Genet*, **2**, 340–342.
13. Bieber, F.R., Brenner, C.H. and Lazer, D. (2006) Human genetics – finding criminals through DNA of their relatives. *Science*, **312**, 1315–1316.
14. Hicks, T., Taroni, F., Curran, J., Buckleton, J., Castella, V. and Ribaux, O. Use of DNA profiles for investigation using a simulated national DNA database: Part II. Statistical and ethical considerations on familial searching. *Forensic Science international. Genetics* 2010 Jan 14. [Epub ahead of print].
15. Harbison, S.A., Hamilton, J.F. and Walsh, S.J. (2001) The New Zealand DNA databank: its development and significance as a crime solving tool. *Science and Justice*, **41**, 33–37.

16. President's DNA Initiative Advancing Justice Through DNA Technology. http://www.dna.gov/ [accessed July 2010].

17. Watch, H.R. (2009) *Testing Justice – The Rape Kit Backlog in Los Angeles City and County*, Human Rights Watch, New York.

18. Williams, R. and Johnson, P. (2005) Forensic DNA Databasing: a European Perspective. Available at: http://www.dur.ac.uk/resources/sass/WilliamsandJohnsonInterimReport2005-1.pdf (accessed 19 April 2010).

19. Schneider, P.M. and Martin, P.D. (2001) Criminal DNA databases: the European situation. *Forensic Science International*, **119**, 232–238.

20. Gill, P., Fereday, L., Morling, N. and Schneider, P.M. (2006) The evolution of DNA databases – recommendations for new European STR loci. *Forensic Science International*, **156**, 242–244.

21. Schneider, P. (2009) Expansion of the European Standard Set of DNA database loci – the current situation. *Profiles in DNA*, **12**, 6–7.

22. Deutsche Welle (2010) Minister pushes for EU-wide DNA data sharing to fight crime. www.dw-world.de/dw/article/0,,2311468,00.html.

11 Kinship testing

The application of DNA profiling to kinship analysis is widespread and offers an easy means of establishing biological relationships. Not surprisingly, paternity testing is the most common form of kinship testing, with hundreds of thousands of tests being performed worldwide each year [1]. Since the first DNA-based kinship test in 1985 [2], DNA analysis has been applied to larger numbers of kinship tests, to the testing of more complex relationships and to the identification of highly compromised human remains.

Parentage testing

PCR-based STR profiling has now become the standard tool and the PowerPlex® 16 (Promega) and AmpFℓSTR® Identifiler® (Applied Biosystems) STR kits that can analyse 15 loci simultaneously are routinely used (see Chapter 6). Laboratories that undertake kinship testing often have over 20 genetic markers at their disposal, including STR markers on the X and Y chromosomes [3, 4] that allow for the testing of complex relationships [5]. SNPs have also been used for parentage testing [6, 7], although this is still uncommon [8].

The sensitivity of STR analysis, although not essential for most forms of paternity testing, allows samples to be routinely collected using buccal swabs [1] and has expanded the possible scenarios where it can be used, for example the analysis of low amounts of DNA recovered from fetal cells [9, 10] (Figure 11.1).

The methodology used to produce DNA profiles for paternity testing is identical to the analysis of material recovered from crime scenes (see Chapters 4–7). However, the interpretation of results is more complex than when comparing profiles from crime scenes and suspects. If the tested child does not possess the alleles that have been inherited from the biological father, we can conclude that he cannot be the biological father. However, because mutations between the father and child could lead to a false exclusion at any given loci [1, 11–14] it is standard practice that an exclusion at three or more loci is required before a test is declared negative.

If we cannot exclude the tested man as being the biological father, then we have to assign a value to indicate the significance of non-exclusion. Likelihood ratios (LRs)

An *Introduction to Forensic Genetics* Second Edition   William Goodwin, Adrian Linacre and Sibte Hadi
© 2011 John Wiley & Sons, Ltd

Figure 11.1 A STR profile generated from fetal cells recovered from amniotic fluid in early pregnancy. In this case it was possible to determine that pregnancy had resulted from a rape, and allowed an informed decision to be made on whether to have the fetus aborted. The profile was generated using the AmpFℓSTR® Profiler Plus® STR kit (Applied Biosystems)

(see Chapter 9), which consider two competing and mutually exclusive hypotheses are used. The hypotheses are:

$$\frac{\text{The tested man is the biological father}}{\text{The tested man is not the biological father}} = \frac{H_p}{H_d}$$

The symbols H_p and H_d were introduced in Chapter 9 when comparing the proposition or hypothesis put forward by the prosecution (H_p) compared with the hypothesis put forward by the defence (H_d). Although in many civil cases the terms prosecution and defence are not appropriate, for continuity and consistency the same terms are used in paternity testing. The result of a LR in this context is called a paternity index (PI) and can be assessed using Equation 11.1.

$$\text{Paternity index} = \frac{\Pr(G_C|G_M, G_{TM}, H_p)}{\Pr(G_C|G_M, G_{TM}, H_d)} \tag{11.1}$$

To calculate this LR, we compare the probability (Pr) of the child's genotype (G_C) given the mother's (G_M) and tested man's genotype (G_{TM}), if the tested man is the biological father (H_p) compared with the probability of the child's genotype given the mother's genotype, if the tested man is not the biological father (H_d).

The numerator and denominator are conditional on the genotypes of the mother, child and tested man. They can be derived using a Punnet square.

Punnett square

The equations are not difficult to understand, particularly if derived from a Punnett square and converted to text form. Consider the case where the mother is genotype (A,B) and child is genotype (B,C) and the tested man is (C,D). If he is the father then the mother must pass on allele B, and the father must pass on allele C. If he is not the father then the mother must still pass on allele B but some other man must pass on allele C. This is given in the Punnett square on the next page.

| | | Alleles from tested man | |
Alleles from mother		C	D
	A	A,C	A,D
	B	**B,C**	B,D

If the tested man **is** the biological father then only one of the four possible combinations match the genotype of the child, therefore we have a probability of 0.25 that the mother and tested man would have a child with the genotype (B,C) (shown in bold).

If the tested man **is not** the biological father then the mother must pass on allele B, which she will do with a probability of 0.5; the probability that a male other than the tested man is the biological father is dependent upon the frequency of allele C (P_c) in the relevant population. The combined probability that this woman and a 'random man' would have a child with the genotype B,C is $0.5 \times P_c$. This gives a LR of:

$$PI = \frac{0.25}{0.5P_c} = \frac{1}{2P_c}$$

The same process can be used for any of the possible combinations. Consider the version where the mother is heterozygous (A,B), the child is heterozygous (A,C) and the tested man is homozygous (C,C).

| | | Alleles from tested man | |
Alleles from mother		C	C
	A	A,C	A,C
	B	B,C	B,C

If the tested man **is** the biological father then there would be a 0.5 probability that the child's genotype would be (A,C), as two of the four combinations are (A,C).

If the tested man **is not** the biological father then the mother must pass on allele A, which she will do with a probability of 0.5; the probability that a male other than the tested man is the biological father is dependent upon the frequency of allele C (P_c) in the relevant population. The combined probability that this woman and a 'random man' would have a child with the genotype A,C is $0.5 \times P_c$. This gives a LR of:

$$PI = \frac{0.5}{0.5P_c} = \frac{1}{P_c}$$

If we consider a final case when the mother is (A,B), the child is (A,B) and the tested man is (A,C).

| | | Alleles from tested man | |
Alleles from mother		A	C
	A	A,A	A,C
	B	A,B	B,C

As with the first example, the numerator (H_p) genotype (A,B) occurs in only one of four ways (0.25). Considering the denominator (H_d): if the mother passed on allele A (probability 0.5) the 'random man' would have to pass on allele B (P_B), the combined probability of these two events is $0.5 \times P_B$; alternatively, the mother could pass on allele B (probability 0.5) and a random man pass on allele A (P_A), with a combined probability of $0.5 \times P_A$. This results in the equation below:

$$PI = \frac{0.25}{0.5P_A + 0.5P_B} = \frac{1}{2(P_A + P_B)}$$

In Table 11.1 all the potential combinations of alleles from a mother, child and tested man are shown along with the resulting numerator, denominator and PI equation.

We can apply the formulae in Table 11.1 to the paternity case that is presented in Table 11.2.

The combined PI is calculated by applying the product rule and multiplying the PI from each locus; in this case the PI is 2 920 823. This can be represented by the statement:

Statement of positive paternity

The results of the DNA testing are 2 920 823 times more likely if the tested man is the biological father of the child than if the biological father is another man, unrelated to the tested man.

In addition to the standard paternity testing where the mother, child and alleged father are available, testing can also be carried out when the mother is not available [12, 18–20]. The formulae used are shown in Table 11.3.

We can apply these formulae to the paternity case shown in Table 11.2 (Table 11.4).

The strength of the PI will naturally vary depending on the given combinations of genotypes in each case. As can be seen from the example above and Figure 11.2 the paternity indices are much lower when the mother is not available for testing.

Probability of paternity

The significance of LRs can be difficult for lay people to evaluate and the results are often presented as a probability of paternity, making the results more accessible. To calculate a probability of paternity requires Bayesian analysis and takes into consideration non-genetic evidence: the LR is multiplied by the prior odds of paternity that is determined by non-genetic evidence, such as the testimony of the woman. It can be calculated using Equation 11.2.

$$\text{Probability of paternity} = \frac{\text{LR} \times \Pr(H_p|\text{non genetic evidence})}{\text{LR} \times \Pr(H_p|\text{non genetic evidence}) + [1 - \Pr(H_p|\text{non genetic evidence})]} \qquad (11.2)$$

Table 11.1 The numerator and denominator that should be used when calculating a paternity index are determined by the genotypes of the child (G_C), mother (G_M) and tested man (G_{TM}). The alleles are represented by A, B, C and D where $A \neq B \neq C \neq D$.

G_C	G_M	G_{TM}	Numerator	Denominator	PI
$A\,A$	$A\,A$	$A\,A$	1	p_A	$\dfrac{1}{p_A}$
		$A\,B$	$1/2$	p_A	$\dfrac{1}{2p_A}$
		$B\,C$	0	p_A	0
	$A\,B$	$A\,A$	$1/2$	$\dfrac{p_A}{2}$	$\dfrac{1}{p_A}$
		$A\,B$	$1/4$	$\dfrac{p_A}{2}$	$\dfrac{1}{2p_A}$
		$A\,C$	$1/4$	$\dfrac{p_A}{2}$	$\dfrac{1}{2p_A}$
		$B\,C$	0	$\dfrac{p_A}{2}$	0
$A\,B$	$A\,A$	$B\,B$	1	P_B	$\dfrac{1}{p_B}$
		$A\,B$	$1/2$	P_B	$\dfrac{1}{2p_B}$
		$B\,C$	$1/2$	P_B	$\dfrac{1}{2p_B}$
		$C\,D$	0	P_B	0
	$A\,B$	$A\,A$	$1/2$	$\dfrac{P_A + P_B}{2}$	$\dfrac{1}{p_A + p_B}$
		$A\,B$	$1/2$	$\dfrac{P_A + P_B}{2}$	$\dfrac{1}{p_A + p_B}$
		$A\,C$	$1/4$	$\dfrac{P_A + P_B}{2}$	$\dfrac{1}{2(p_A + p_B)}$
		$B\,C$	$1/4$	$\dfrac{P_A + P_B}{2}$	$\dfrac{1}{2(p_A + p_B)}$
		$C\,D$	0	$\dfrac{P_A + P_B}{2}$	0
	$A\,C$	$B\,B$	$1/2$	$\dfrac{P_B}{2}$	$\dfrac{1}{p_B}$
		$A\,B$	$1/4$	$\dfrac{P_B}{2}$	$\dfrac{1}{2p_B}$
		$B\,C$	$1/4$	$\dfrac{P_B}{2}$	$\dfrac{1}{2p_B}$
		$B\,D$	$1/4$	$\dfrac{P_B}{2}$	$\dfrac{1}{2p_B}$
		$C\,D$	0	$\dfrac{P_B}{2}$	0

Based on Lucy [15], p. 174 and Evett and Weir [16], p. 168.

Table 11.2 The result of a paternity test using the Powerplex® 16 STR Kit (Promega). The alleles that the child could have inherited from the mother are underlined and the paternal alleles are shown in bold. The A, B, C and D symbols correspond to symbols in Table 11.1

Locus	Child (G_C)	Mother (G_M)	Tested man (G_{TM})	Num	Denom	PI	$P_{i/j}$	PI
D3S1358	$\underline{15}^A - \mathbf{15}^A$	$14^B - \underline{15}^A$	$\mathbf{15}^A - 19^C$	$1/4$	$\dfrac{P_A}{2}$	$\dfrac{1}{2p_A}$	0.3239	1.54
VWA	$17^B - \underline{18}^A$	$16^C - \underline{18}^A$	$\mathbf{17}^B - 18^A$	$1/4$	$\dfrac{P_B}{2}$	$\dfrac{1}{2p_B}$	0.2715	1.84
D16S359	$\underline{11}^A - \mathbf{12}^B$	$\underline{11}^A - 13^C$	$\mathbf{12}^B - 13^C$	$1/4$	$\dfrac{P_B}{2}$	$\dfrac{1}{2p_B}$	0.2773	1.80
D8S1179	$\underline{10}^A - \underline{13}^B$	$\underline{10}^A - \underline{13}^B$	$\mathbf{10}^A - 10^A$	$1/2$	$\dfrac{P_A + P_B}{2}$	$\dfrac{1}{p_A + p_B}$	0.0630 0.3033	2.73
D21S11	$\underline{30}^A - \mathbf{32.2}^B$	$\underline{30}^A - 31^C$	$27^D - \mathbf{32.2}^B$	$1/4$	$\dfrac{P_B}{2}$	$\dfrac{1}{2p_B}$	0.1245	4.02
D18S51	$\underline{13}^A - \underline{14}^B$	$\underline{13}^A - \underline{14}^B$	$12^C - \mathbf{14}^B$	$1/4$	$\dfrac{P_A + P_B}{2}$	$\dfrac{1}{2(p_A + p_B)}$	0.1326 0.2063	1.48
THO1	$\underline{9}^A - \mathbf{9.3}^B$	$\underline{9}^A - \underline{9.3}^B$	$6^C - \mathbf{9.3}^B$	$1/4$	$\dfrac{P_A + P_B}{2}$	$\dfrac{1}{2(p_A + p_B)}$	0.1407 0.2624	1.24
FGA	$\underline{18}^A - \mathbf{23}^B$	$\underline{18}^A - 25^C$	$\mathbf{23}^B - 23^B$	$1/2$	$\dfrac{P_B}{2}$	$\dfrac{1}{p_B}$	0.1440	6.94
D13S317	$\underline{8}^A - \mathbf{13}^B$	$\underline{8}^A - 11^C$	$11^C - \mathbf{13}^B$	$1/4$	$\dfrac{P_B}{2}$	$\dfrac{1}{2p_B}$	0.1444	3.46
CSF1PO	$\underline{11}^A - \mathbf{11}^A$	$\underline{11}^A - 13^B$	$\mathbf{11}^A - 13^B$	$1/4$	$\dfrac{P_A}{2}$	$\dfrac{1}{2p_A}$	0.2916	1.71
D7S820	$\underline{9}^A - \mathbf{9}^A$	$\underline{9}^A - 10^B$	$\mathbf{9}^A - 11^C$	$1/4$	$\dfrac{P_A}{2}$	$\dfrac{1}{2p_A}$	0.0998	5.01
TPOX	$8^B - \underline{10}^A$	$\underline{10}^A - 11^C$	$\mathbf{8}^B - 8^B$	$1/2$	$\dfrac{P_B}{2}$	$\dfrac{1}{p_B}$	0.5243	1.91
D5S818	$\underline{11}^A - \underline{12}^B$	$\underline{11}^A - \underline{12}^B$	$\mathbf{11}^A - 12^B$	$1/2$	$\dfrac{P_A + P_B}{2}$	$\dfrac{1}{p_A + p_B}$	0.3618 0.2992	1.51
Penta D	$\mathbf{13}^B - \underline{15}^A$	$12^C - \underline{15}^A$	$12^D - \mathbf{13}^B$	$1/4$	$\dfrac{P_B}{2}$	$\dfrac{1}{2p_B}$	0.1726	2.90
Penta E	$\underline{10}^A - \mathbf{18}^B$	$\underline{10}^A - 10^A$	$16^C - \mathbf{18}^B$	$1/2$	P_B	$\dfrac{1}{2p_B}$	0.0304	16.4
						Combined PI		**2 920 823**

The allele frequencies were taken from Marino *et al.* [17].

Taking the above paternity test it is possible to turn the LR into a probability of paternity for any prior odds of paternity; for example:

Table 11.3 Formulae used to calculate paternity indices in cases where no mother is available for testing. The alleles are represented by A, B and C where $A \neq B \neq C$ [21]

G_C	G_{TM}	PI
$A\,A$	$A\,A$	$\dfrac{1}{p_A}$
	$A\,B$	$\dfrac{1}{2p_A}$
$A\,B$	$A\,A$	$\dfrac{1}{2p_A}$
	$B\,B$	$\dfrac{1}{2p_B}$
	$A\,B$	$\dfrac{p_A + p_B}{4p_Ap_B}$
	$A\,C$	$\dfrac{1}{4p_A}$

Prior probability $= 0.1$

$$\text{Probability of paternity} = \frac{2\,920\,823 \times 0.1}{(2\,920\,823 \times 0.1) + (1 - 0.1)} = 0.999996919$$

When this figure is used to report the results of a test it is often quoted as a percentage, which is more accessible to non-scientists. In this case the probability of paternity would be quoted as 99.9997%.

The value that is attributed to the prior odds of paternity is, of course, subjective. In civil cases, the value of 0.5 is commonly used, although there is little scientific merit to this value. In criminal cases, probabilities of paternity are often not presented because it is the duty of the jury/judge to assess the prior odds of paternity. If results are presented as a probability of paternity, a range of values calculated using different prior odds is often quoted (Table 11.5).

With low paternity indices the impact of prior odds can be significant. However, with the possibility of analysing a large number of STR loci, the PIs are typically in the millions and the posterior probability of paternity is therefore extremely high, even when the prior odds are very low. In the paternity test presented above, even with the prior odds as low as 0.001, the probability of paternity is still 99.9966%.

Calculations of paternity indices can also incorporate correction factors to allow for mutations and silent alleles [21] and also deficiencies in allele frequency databases;

Table 11.4 With the mother's genotype from the paternity case shown in Table 11.2 we can recalculate the paternity index for what is now a motherless case. The results, while still providing very strong support for paternity, are approximately 28-fold weaker than when the mother was available for testing

Locus	Child (G_C)	Tested man (G_{TM})	PI	$P_{A/B}$	PI
D3S1358	$15^A - 15^A$	$15^A - 19^B$	$\dfrac{1}{2p_A}$	0.3239	1.54
vWA	$17^A - 18^B$	$17^A - 18^B$	$\dfrac{p_A + p_B}{4p_Ap_B}$	0.2715 / 0.1816	2.30
D16S359	$11^B - 12^A$	$12^A - 13^C$	$\dfrac{1}{4p_A}$	0.2773	0.90
D8S1179	$10^A - 13^B$	$10^A - 10^A$	$\dfrac{1}{2p_A}$	0.0630	7.94
D21S11	$30^B - 32.2^A$	$27^C - 32.2^A$	$\dfrac{1}{4p_A}$	0.1245	2.01
D18S51	$13^B - 14^A$	$12^C - 14^A$	$\dfrac{1}{4p_A}$	0.2063	1.21
TH01	$9^B - 9.3^A$	$6^C - 9.3^A$	$\dfrac{1}{4p_A}$	0.2624	0.95
FGA	$18^B - 23^A$	$23^A - 23^A$	$\dfrac{1}{2p_A}$	0.1440	3.47
D13S317	$8^B - 13^A$	$11^C - 13^A$	$\dfrac{1}{4p_A}$	0.1444	1.73
CSF1PO	$11^A - 11^A$	$11^A - 13^B$	$\dfrac{1}{2p_A}$	0.2916	1.71
D7S820	$9^A - 9^A$	$9^A - 11^B$	$\dfrac{1}{2p_A}$	0.0998	5.01
TPOX	$8^A - 10^B$	$8^A - 8^A$	$\dfrac{1}{2p_B}$	0.5243	1.91
D5S818	$11^A - 12^B$	$11^A - 12^B$	$\dfrac{p_A + p_B}{4p_Ap_B}$	0.3618 / 0.2992	1.53
Penta D	$13^A - 15^B$	$12^C - 13^A$	$\dfrac{1}{4p_A}$	0.1726	1.45
Penta E	$10^B - 18^A$	$16^C - 18^A$	$\dfrac{1}{4p_A}$	0.0304	8.22
			Combined PI		104 759

in particular, the effects of subpopulations [3, 8, 21–23]. Fortunately, computer programs have been developed to deal with both routine and complex scenarios [24–30].

This chapter so far has discussed paternity testing. Needless to say, on rare occasions there is also the need to undertake maternity testing. The same principles and methods apply. In addition to parentage testing, more complex relationships can be

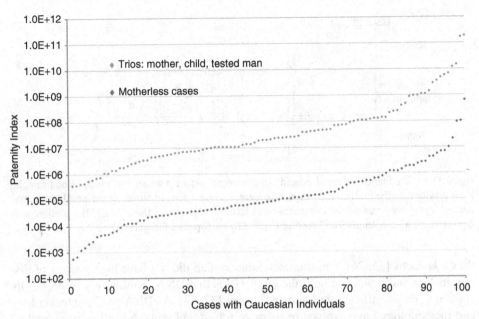

Figure 11.2 Paternity indices are shown for 100 trio (mother, child and tested man) and 100 motherless paternity cases using the PowerPlex® 16 loci. The cases were simulated – values for trio and motherless cases were based on different simulations

Table 11.5 The impact of prior probabilities on the probability of paternity is shown with two paternity indexes: one with a value of 1000 and the other taken from the above example, with a value of 2 920 823

	Paternity index	
Prior odds	1000	2 920 823
0.0001	0.090 917 356	0.996 588 329
0.0010	0.500 250 125	0.999 658 09
0.0100	0.909 918 107	0.999 966 107
0.1000	0.991 080 278	0.999 996 919
0.5000	0.999 000 999	0.999 999 658
0.7500	0.999 666 778	0.999 999 886
0.9000	0.999 888 901	0.999 999 962

examined than those encountered in parentage testing, such as determination of sibship [31] and paternity tests to discriminate between close relatives [16, 32–34].

Identification of human remains

The first application of DNA analysis to the identification of human remains was in 1987, when skeletal remains were profiled using single nucleotide polymorphisms in

Figure 11.3 The identification of human remains recovered from an air crash [40]. Blood samples were provided by the mother and father who were missing a son. In alleles in the profile of human remains could have come from the mother and father (indicated by the arrows). The profiles were generated using the AmpFℓSTR® Profiler Plus® STR kit (Applied Biosystems)

the DQα locus [35, 36]. Unfortunately, this system did not have high powers of discrimination and it was not until the early 1990s that DNA profiling was successfully applied to the identification of human remains [37, 38]. As DNA profiling technology and methodology have evolved to be more robust and powerful, it has been applied to increasingly complex situations including the identification of people killed in air crashes [28, 39–42]; fire [43–46]; terrorist attacks [47–50]; natural disasters [51]; and war [52–55]. STRs are the most commonly used tool but mitochondrial DNA (see Chapter 13) and SNPs (see Chapter 12) have also been employed on occasion.

The matching of human remains can be through comparison of DNA recovered from personal objects that belonged to the missing person, such as combs and toothbrushes [56], or by comparison to close family members (Figure 11.3).

In cases that involve hundreds of victims, the statistical analysis becomes very complex. Because of the high number of pair-wise comparisons that are made between the victims and relatives, the potential for coincidental matches that result in false positives and ultimately misidentifications is significant [51, 56, 57]. The existence of relatives within the population of victims also complicates the analysis [28, 51] and there are limitations as to what can be achieved.

Further reading

Balding, D.J. (2005) *Weight-of-evidence for Forensic DNA Profiles*, John Wiley & Sons, Ltd, Chichester, pp. 82–134.

Buckleton, J., Triggs, C.M. and Walsh, S.J. (2005) *Forensic DNA Evidence Interpretation*, CRC Press, pp. 341–347.

References

1. American Association of Blood Banks (2004) Annual Report Summary for Testing in 2004.
2. Jeffreys, A.J., Brookfield, J.F.Y. and Semenoff, R. (1985) Positive identification of an immigration test-case using human DNA fingerprints. *Nature*, **317**, 818–819.

3. Szibor, R., Krawczak, M., Hering, S., Edelmann, J., Kuhlisch, E. and Krause, D. (2003) Use of X-linked markers for forensic purposes. *International Journal of Legal Medicine*, **117**, 67–74.

4. Hatsch, D., Keyser, C., Hienne, R. and Bertrand, L. (2007) Resolving paternity relationships using X-chromosome STRs and Bayesian networks. *Journal of Forensic Sciences*, **52**, 895–897.

5. Junge, A., Brinkmann, B., Fimmers, R. and Madea, B. (2006) Mutations or exclusion: an unusual case in paternity testing. *International Journal of Legal Medicine*, **120**, 360–363.

6. Borsting, C., Sanchez, J.J., Hansen, H.E., Hansen, A.J., Bruun, H.Q. and Morling, N. (2008) Performance of the SNPforID 52 SNP-plex assay in paternity testing. *Forensic Science International: Genetics*, **2**, 292–300.

7. Phillips, C., Fondevila, M., Garcia-Magarinos, A., Rodriguez, A., Salas, A. and Carracedo, A. (2008) Resolving relationship tests that show ambiguous STR results using autosomal SNPs as supplementary markers. *Forensic Science International: Genetics*, **2**, 198–204.

8. Thomsen, A.R., Hallenberg, C., Simonsen, B.T., Langkjaer, R.B. and Morling, N. (2009) A report of the 2002–2008 paternity testing workshops of the English speaking working group of the international society for forensic genetics. *Forensic Science International: Genetics*, **3**, 214–221.

9. Makrydimas, G., Georgiou, I., Bouba, I., Lolis, D. and Nicolaides, K.H. (2004) Early prenatal diagnosis by celocentesis. *Ultrasound in Obstetrics and Gynecology*, **23**, 482–485.

10. Makrydimas, G., Georgiou, I., Kranas, V., Kaponis, A. and Lolis, D. (2004) Prenatal paternity testing using DNA extracted from coelomic cells. *Fetal Diagnosis and Therapy*, **19**, 75–77.

11. Brinkmann, B., Klintschar, M., Neuhuber, F., Huhne, J. and Rolf, B. (1998) Mutation rate in human microsatellites: influence of the structure and length of the tandem repeat. *American Journal of Human Genetics*, **62**, 1408–1415.

12. Chakraborty, R., Jin, L. and Zhong, Y.X. (1994) Paternity evaluation in cases lacking a mother and nondetectable alleles. *International Journal of Legal Medicine*, **107**, 127–131.

13. Gunn, P.R., Trueman, K., Stapleton, P. and Klarkowski, D.B. (1997) DNA analysis in disputed parentage: the occurrence of two apparently false exclusions of paternity, both at short tandem repeat (STR) loci, in the one child. *Electrophoresis*, **18**, 1650–1652.

14. Leopoldino, A.M. and Pena, S.D.J. (2003) The mutational spectrum of human autosomal tetranucleotide microsatellites. *Human Mutation*, **21**, 71–79.

15. Lucy, D. (2005) *Introduction to Statistics for Forensic Scientists*, John Wiley & Sons, Ltd, Chichester.

16. Evett, I.W. and Weir, B.S. (1998) *Interpreting DNA Evidence*, Sinauer Associates, Inc.

17. Marino, M., Sala, A. and Corach, D. (2006) Population genetic analysis of 15 autosomal STRs loci in the central region of Argentina. *Forensic Science International*, **161**, 72–77.

18. Brenner, C.H. (1993) A note on paternity computation in cases lacking a mother. *Transfusion*, **33**, 51–54.

19. Poetsch, M., Ludcke, C., Repenning, A., Fischer, L., Malyusz, V., Simeoni, E. *et al.* (2006) The problem of single parent/child paternity analysis – practical results involving 336 children and 348 unrelated men. *Forensic Science International*, **159**, 98–103.

20. Thomson, J.A., Ayres, K.L., Pilotti, V., Barrett, M.N., Walker, J.I.H., Debenham, P.G. *et al.* (2001) Analysis of disputed single-parent/child and sibling relationships using 16 STR loci. *International Journal of Legal Medicine*, **115**, 128–134.

21. Buckleton, J., Triggs, C.M. and Walsh, S.J. (2005) *Forensic DNA Evidence Interpretation*, CRC Press, Boca Raton, pp. 341–437.

22. Ayres, K.L. (2000) Relatedness testing in subdivided populations. *Forensic Science International*, **114**, 107–115.

23. Fung, W.K., Carracedo, A. and, Y.Q. (2003) Testing for kinship in a subdivided population. *Forensic Science International*, **135**, 105–109.

24. Brenner, C.H. DNAVIEW. http://dna-view.com/dnaview.htm (accessed July 2010).

25. Brenner, C.H. (1997) Symbolic kinship program. *Genetics*, **145**, 535–542.

26. Fung, W.K. (2003) User-friendly programs for easy calculations in paternity testing and kinship determinations. *Forensic Science International*, **136**, 22–34.

27. Fung, W.K., Hu, Y.Q. and Chung, Y.K. (2006) On statistical analysis of forensic DNA: theory, methods and computer programs. *Forensic Science International*, **162**, 17–23.

28. Leclair, B., Fregeau, C.J., Bowen, K.L. and Fourney, R.M. (2004) Enhanced kinship analysis and STR-based DNA typing for human identification in mass fatality incidents: the Swissair Flight 111 disaster. *Journal of Forensic Sciences*, **49**, 939–953.

29. Riancho, J.A. and Zarrabeitia, M.T. (2003) A Windows-based software for common paternity and sibling analyses. *Forensic Science International*, **135**, 232–234.

30. Drabek, J. (2009) Validation of software for calculating the likelihood ratio for parentage and kinship. *Forensic Science International: Genetics*, **3**, 112–118.

31. Wenk, R.E., Traver, M. and Chiafari, F.A. (1996) Determination of sibship in any two persons. *Transfusion*, **36**, 259–262.

32. Ayres, K.L. and Balding, D.J. (2005) Paternity index calculations when some individuals share common ancestry. *Forensic Science International*, **151**, 101–103.

33. Fung, W.K., Chung, Y.K. and Wong, D.M. (2002) Power of exclusion revisited: probability of excluding relatives of the true father from paternity. *International Journal of Legal Medicine*, **116**, 64–67.

34. Wenk, R.E. and Chiafari, F.A. (2000) Distinguishing full siblings from half-siblings in limited pedigrees. *Transfusion*, **40**, 44–47.

35. Blake, E., Crim, D., Mihalovich, J., Higuchi, R., Walsh, P.S. and Erlich, H. (1992) Polymerase chain-reaction (PCR) amplification and human-leukocyte antigen (HLA)-DQ-alpha oligonucleotide typing on biological evidence samples – casework experience. *Journal of Forensic Sciences*, **37**, 700–726.

36. Stoneking, M., Hedgecock, D., Higuchi, R.G., Vigilant, L. and Erlich, H.A. (1991) Population variation of human mtDNA control region sequences detected by enzymatic amplification and sequence-specific oligonucleotide probes. *American Journal of Human Genetics*, **48**, 370–382.

37. Hagelberg, E., Gray, I.C. and Jeffreys, A.J. (1991) Identification of the skeletal remains of a murder victim by DNA analysis. *Nature*, **352**, 427–429.

38. Sajantila, A., Strom, M., Budowle, B., Karhunen, P.J. and Peltonen, L. (1991) The polymerase chain-reaction and postmortem forensic identity testing – application of amplified D1S80 and HLA-DQ-alpha loci to the identification of fire victims. *Forensic Science International*, **51**, 23–34.

39. Ballantyne, J. (1997) Mass disaster genetics. *Nature Genetics*, **15**, 329–331.

40. Goodwin, W., Linacre, A. and Vanezis, P. (1999) The use of mitochondrial DNA and short tandem repeat typing in the identification of air crash victims. *Electrophoresis*, **20**, 1707–1711.

41. Hsu, C.M., Huang, N.E., Tsai, L.C., Kao, L.G., Chao, C.H., Linacre, A. *et al.* (1999) Identification of victims of the 1998 Taoyuan airbus crash accident using DNA analysis. *International Journal of Legal Medicine*, **113**, 43–46.

42. Olaisen, B., Stenersen, M. and Mevag, B. (1997) Identification by DNA analysis of the victims of the August 1996 Spitsbergen civil aircraft disaster. *Nature Genetics*, **15**, 402–405.

43. Calacal, G.C., Delfin, F.C., Tan, M.M.M., Roewer, L., Magtanong, D.L. and Lara, M.C. (2005) Identification of exhumed remains of fire tragedy victims using conventional methods and autosomal/Y-chromosomal short tandem repeat DNA profiling. *American Journal of Forensic Medicine and Pathology*, **26**, 285–291.

44. Clayton, T.M., Whitaker, J.P., Fisher, D.L., Lee, D.A., Holland, M.M., Weedn, V.W. *et al.* (1995) Further validation of a quadruplex STR DNA typing system: a collaborative effort to identify victims of a mass disaster. *Forensic Science International*, **76**, 17–25.

45. Clayton, T.M., Whitaker, J.P. and Maguire, C.N. (1995) Identification of bodies from the scene of a mass disaster using DNA amplification of short tandem repeat (STR) loci. *Forensic Science International*, **76**, 7–15.

46. Meyer, H.J. (2003) The Kaprun cable car fire disaster – aspects of forensic organisation following a mass fatality with 155 victims. *Forensic Science International*, **138**, 1–7.

47. Budimlija, Z.M., Prinz, M.K., Zelson-Mundorff, A., Wiersema, J., Bartelink, E., MacKinnon, G. *et al.* (2003) World trade center human identification project: experiences with individual body identification cases. *Croatian Medical Journal*, **44**, 259–263.

48. Budowle, B., Bieber F.R., Eisenberg A.J. (2005) Forensic aspects of mass disasters: strategic considerations for DNA-based human identification. *Legal Medicine*, **7**, 230–243.

49. Holland, M.M., Cave. C.A., Holland, C.A. and Bille, T.W. (2003) Development of a quality, high throughput DNA analysis procedure for skeletal samples to assist with the identification of victims from the world trade center attacks. *Croatian Medical Journal*, **44**, 264–272.

50. Kahana, T., Freund, M. and Hiss, J. (1997) Suicidal terrorist bombings in Israel - identification of human remains. *Journal of Forensic Sciences*, **42**, 260–264.

51. Brenner, C.H. (2006) Some mathematical problems in the DNA identification of victims in the 2004 tsunami and similar mass fatalities. *Forensic Science International*, **157**, 172–180.

52. Boles, T.C., Snow, C.C. and Stover, E. (1995) Forensic DNA testing on skeletal remains from mass graves – a pilot project in Guatemala. *Journal of Forensic Sciences*, **40**, 349–355.

53. Holland, M.M., Fisher, D.L., Mitchell, L.G., Rodriguez, W.C., Canik, J.J., Merril, C.R. *et al.* (1993) Mitochondrial-DNA sequence-analysis of human skeletal remains – identification of remains from the Vietnam-war. *Journal of Forensic Sciences*, **38**, 542–553.

54. Huffine, E., Crews, J., Kennedy, B., Bomberger, K. and Zinbo, A. (2001) Mass identification of persons missing from the break-up of the former Yugoslavia: structure, function, and role of the International Commission on Missing Persons. *Croatian Medical Journal*, **42**, 271–275.

55. Lleonart, R., Riego, E., de la Pena, M.V.S., Bacallao, K., Amaro, F., Santiesteban, M. *et al.* (2000) Forensic identification of skeletal remains from members of Ernesto Che Guevara's guerrillas in Bolivia based an DNA typing. *International Journal of Legal Medicine*, **113**, 98–101.

56. Brenner, C.H. and Weir, B.S. (2003) Issues and strategies in the DNA identification of World Trade Center victims. *Theoretical Population Biology*, **63**, 173–178.

57. Gornik, I., Marcikic, M., Kubat, M., Primorac, D. and Lauc, G. (2002) The identification of war victims by reverse paternity is associated with significant risks of false inclusion. *International Journal of Legal Medicine*, **116**, 255–257.

12 Single nucleotide polymorphisms

One of the most significant outcomes of the Human Genome Project has been the identification of large numbers of SNPs [1–3]. The application of SNPs to forensic analysis is currently limited to some specialist cases. However, with advances both in our knowledge of SNPs and in the technology used to detect the polymorphisms, SNP analysis may play an increasingly important role in the future.

SNPs – occurrence and structure

'SNPs are single base pair positions in genomic DNA at which different sequence alternatives (alleles) exist in normal individuals in some population(s), wherein the least frequent allele has an abundance of 1% or greater' [4]. The structure of a SNP is very simple, an example is shown in Figure 12.1.

Initial sequencing of the human genome identified over 2 million SNPs [5, 6]. Following the first drafts of the human genome, the International HapMap Project was established in 2001 to catalogue common patterns of sequence variation, using populations that represented four geographical regions (Europe, sub-Saharan Africa (Nigeria) and Southeast Asia (China and Japan) [7]. The second phase of the project has characterized over 3.1 million SNPs in 270 individuals from the geographically diverse populations [8]. Other databases contain additional SNPs: the National Center for Biotechnology Information SNP database (NCBI dbSNP) reports over 10 million validated SNPs [9, 10]. Whole genome sequencing of individuals' genomes has shown that they contain around 3–4 million SNPs relative to the NCBI's reference human genome [11–16].

Forensic value of SNPs

Given the array of SNPs available in the genome, and with individuals differing at millions of positions, the potential for SNPs to discriminate between individuals is enormous. As SNPs are biallelic the population falls in to one of three types. Given the example in Figure 12.1 everyone would be one of CC, CT or TT. This type of polymorphism intrinsically limits the information that can be gained from the analysis

An Introduction to Forensic Genetics Second Edition William Goodwin, Adrian Linacre and Sibte Hadi
© 2011 John Wiley & Sons, Ltd

Figure 12.1 SNPs are created when the DNA replication enzymes make a mistake as they copy the cell's DNA during meiosis. The enzyme incorporates the wrong nucleotide approximately once every $2–3 \times 10^8$ bases. In the vast majority of cases SNPs are biallelic and only have two different alleles. In the alleles shown above, the thymine nucleotide has been replaced by a cytosine. This is a transition as a pyrimidine has been altered for another pyrimidine. A transversions occurs when a pyrimidine (or purine) is change for a purine (pyrimidine)

of any given SNP, and this has been the major factor limiting their application to forensic analysis: between 50 and 80 SNPs are required to achieve the same levels of discrimination as the current STR-based methods [17, 18]. The technology used for SNP detection is evolving and SNP analysis is becoming possible in many forensic laboratories.

Detection of SNPs

There are many techniques available for the resolution of SNPs. In the 1970s it was established that particular enzymes produced by bacteria can be used to cut the DNA molecule by recognizing specific sequences [19]. Restriction digestion can be used to genotype SNPs when the SNP either creates or destroys a particular restriction enzyme recognition sequence [20, 21], but the method is limited for forensic casework because it needs a large amount of DNA and is a long and laborious process.

Sanger sequencing

Sanger sequencing, also known as chain-termination sequencing, was developed in the late 1970s and is a milestone in the development of molecular biology [22]. The sequencing takes advantage of the biochemistry of DNA replication. The first stage of the analysis is to amplify the target region using PCR; amplified products are then used as the template in a sequencing reaction. The DNA sequencing reaction is similar to PCR amplification and the reaction mixture is very similar, containing the thermophilic *Taq* DNA polymerase and deoxynucleotide triphosphates (dNTPs). It differs from PCR in that only one primer is used and, in addition to the dNTPs, there are four fluorescently labelled dideoxyribonucleotide triphosphates (ddNTPs); each ddNTP is labelled with a different coloured dye [23]. The ddNTPs do not contain the hydroxyl group on the 3′ carbon, which prevents any extension of the DNA molecule [24] (Figure 12.2).

Figure 12.2 A primer anneals to the template strand. This is extended by *Taq* polymerase until a ddNTP is incorporated. The ddNTPs are incorporated at random which leads to a collection of extension molecules that differ from each other by one nucleotide (shown above labelled 1–8). The four ddNTPs are labelled with different fluorescent dyes that are detected during capillary electrophoresis

Figure 12.3 The sequence of a region of the mitochondrial genome. The sequencing software interprets the sequence data and 'calls' the bases and this information is provided above the sequencing peaks

The concentration of dNTPs is higher than ddNTPs and therefore in most cases a dNTP is added. The ddNTPs are incorporated at random intervals along the molecule. This produces a range of different sized molecules. The products of the sequencing reaction are analysed using capillary gel electrophoresis systems, such as the ABI PRISM® 310 Genetic Analyzer, which separates DNA to single base pair resolution and can simultaneously detect four different fluorescent labels (Figure 12.3).

Sequencing is not a practical option for the analysis of SNPs in a forensic context. Most SNPs are widely dispersed around the genome and a separate reaction would be required for each SNP. An exception is the mitochondrial genome, where a number of SNPs are concentrated into a small area and can be analysed in a small number of reactions (see Chapter 13). Sequencing has also been a powerful method to type SNPs within rapidly evolving regions of DNA in the HIV virus [25, 26].

SNP detection for forensic applications

Restriction digestion and sequence analysis are not viable methods to use for most forensic cases that might require the analysis of 50–80 SNPs dispersed around the genome. A number of methods have evolved that can be applied to the detection of multiple SNPs. Methods that are based around the concepts of either primer extension or primer hybridization are the most widely used.

Primer extension

Primer extension is a robust method for discriminating between different alleles and several methodologies have been developed [27]. One of the commonly used methods is the mini-sequencing reaction [28]. The basis of the reaction is very similar to Sanger sequencing. The first part of the procedure is to amplify the target region using PCR. An internal primer then anneals to the denatured PCR product; the 3′ end of the primer is adjacent to the polymorphic site. The primer is then extended by *Taq* polymerase but only ddNTPs that are labelled with fluorescent dyes are provided, therefore the primer is only extended by one nucleotide. The extended primer can be analysed using capillary gel electrophoresis and the colour of the detected peak allows the SNP to be characterized (Figure 12.4). The widely used SNaPshot® kit (Applied Biosystems) is based on this methodology.

By using different sized primers and different fluorescent tags for each of the four bases, a large number of SNPs can be simultaneously detected [29].

Variations on the primer extension technique include pyrosequencing [30, 31]; microarrays, where the extension primers are attached to a silicon chip [32, 33]; and allele-specific extension, when the primer is only extended if it is 100% complementary to the target sequence [34].

Allele-specific hybridization

Under stringent conditions, even one nucleotide mismatching between a template and primer can differentiate between two alleles (Figure 12.5).

There is a large number of methods that exploit the hybridization of probes, including Taqman® MGB (minor groove binder) assays [35], GenPlex [36], reverse dot blots [37]; LightCycler® assays [38]; molecular beacons [3, 39, 40]; and GeneChips® [41] (see Ref. [27] for details).

(a)

5'-TGCATCGTCACGTGACTGCTAGTCAAT - 3' Template
TGCACTGACGATCAGTTA - 5' Primer

(b)

SBE

(c)

Figure 12.4 The primer extension assay. (a) The target sequence is amplified using PCR and the products are used as the template in the extension assay; (b) an internal primer hybridizes to the target adjacent to the SNP and a single fluorescently labelled ddNTP is added by *Taq* polymerase; (c) the labelled single-base extension (SBE) product is analysed using capillary electrophoresis

(a)   (b)

Figure 12.5 Allele-specific hybridization: allele-specific oligonucleotide (ASO) probes that include the SNP are hybridized with the target DNA. (a) Under highly stringent conditions only perfectly matched sequences will form stable interactions and (b) with one mismatch in sequence the ASO will not hybridize

Forensic applications of SNPs

A vast amount of data is available on the different SNPs in the human genome and one of the biggest tasks when applying SNPs to forensic applications is to select the most appropriate SNPs from the overwhelming numbers that are available. The choice of SNPs is very much dependent on the application. The characteristics that a SNP must fulfil are that they need to be polymorphic, that is with not one allele being very common and the other very rare, and that they can be examined at the same in a multiplex similar to that for STR loci.

Forensic identification

The vast majority of forensic DNA analysis involves the characterization of biological material recovered from the scene of a crime. Several panels of SNPs have been developed that are designed to provide maximum discrimination powers for forensic identification [29, 42, 43]. These contain SNPs that are polymorphic in all major population groups. A panel containing 52 SNPs was developed by the SNPforID Consortium [29]. Using this panel of SNPs produced match probabilities that ranged from 5.0×10^{-19} in an Asian population to 5.0×10^{-21} in a European population. When applied to paternity testing, average paternity indices of between 336 000 in Asian populations and 550 000 in European populations were achieved.

However, even with the high discrimination power, the effort involved in analysing 50 SNPs is greater than when undertaking standard STR analysis. The major attractions of using SNPs with the current technology is that SNP analysis can provide results from highly degraded DNA when conventional STR profiling has failed [42, 44] and also the low mutation rate of SNPs.

Prediction of the geographical ancestry

In many cases, the identification of the population group from which a crime scene sample has come from can be valuable intelligence for the investigating agencies: was the person who left the material at the crime scene of Caucasian, Asian, African, mixed ancestry? Panels consisting of mtDNA SNPs and Y SNPs have already been found useful for this purpose [45, 46] but are intrinsically limited by the fact that they can only provide information on either the maternal or paternal ancestry. Autosomal SNPs that have different frequencies in different major population groups can provide valuable information on geographic ancestry [47, 48]. Many of the SNPs selected for this purpose are associated with coding regions that have been subjected to selection pressures. These include pigmentation genes and genes involved with the metabolism of xenobiotics. The pigmentation genes, in addition to providing information on geographic ancestry, can also give information on phenotype of the person who deposited the biological material at a crime scene, including skin, hair and eye colour [49–52].

SNPs compared with STR loci

Current STR-based multiplex kits like AmpFℓSTR® Identifiler® and PowerPlex® 16 can amplify 15 STR loci and the amelogenin locus. Using the current technology it is difficult to co-amplify and detect any more STR loci. Also, the size of the amplicon for each STR is quite large. The great advantage STRs have over SNPs is their power

Table 12.1 A comparison of the properties of SNPs and STRs

	STR	SNP
Frequency of occurrence	Once every 15 kb	Once every 500 bp
Typical rate of mutation	10^{-3}	$2-3 \times 10^{-8}$
Typical number of alleles	Between 5 and 20	2
Potential to multiplex	Currently 15 STR loci examined in one reaction	Difficult to amplify more than 50 SNPs in one reaction
Number of loci required to have a P_M of 1 in 1 billion	10	~60
Method of detection	Capillary gel electrophoresis (CGE)	CGE, microarrays, mass spectroscopy
Automation potential	Medium	High
Artefacts	Amplification of STRs can produce artefacts such as stutter and split peaks	No stutter artefacts associated with the amplification of the SNPs
Amount of DNA required	~0.5 ng–1 ng	~100 pg
Size of amplicon	Amplicon sizes typically between 100 bp and 400 bp	Amplicon sizes can be less than 100 bp
Mixtures	Interpretation of mixtures of STR loci is possible	Mixtures of SNP loci can be highly problematic to interpret
Predicting geographical origin	Limited ethnic identification from STR loci	Some SNPs can be associated with particular ethnic groups
Phenotypic information	No possibility to infer phenotype	Possible to predict some hair colour, eye colour, skin colour

of discrimination due to the large number of alleles they have in comparison with biallelic SNPs. In contrast to STRs, around four times more SNPs are required to reach the discrimination power equivalent to STR loci. Another major disadvantage to using SNPs is that mixtures of two or more people might be either problematic or impossible to interpret since SNPs are biallelic markers. In addition, current DNA databases consist of profiles comprising STR loci and therefore SNPs cannot be used in that context. At the same time it is possible to analyse hundreds of SNP loci and, because of their structure, the amplicon size can be much smaller, typically less than 100 bp. This allows the detection of DNA templates that are highly degraded and may generate data when standard STR typing fails to generate a result. A comparison between STR and SNP markers is shown in Table 12.1.

In the foreseeable future, STRs will be the most commonly used genetic polymorphism analysed. They are tried and tested in most judicial systems and also form the basis of most forensic DNA databases. Even so, the use of SNPs in forensic genetics is likely to increase in the coming years and may at some point in the future replace the analysis of STR polymorphisms. The application of SNPs to specialized applications, for example SNP-based blood grouping [43, 53] and molecular autopsy (looking for mutations that can explain sudden death [54, 55]), is likely to become more widespread.

References

1. Miller, R.D., Phillips, M.S., Jo, I., Donaldson, M.A., Studebaker, J.F., Addleman, N. *et al.* (2005) High-density single-nucleotide polymorphism maps of the human genome. *Genomics*, **86**, 117–126.
2. Sachidanandam, R., Weissman, D., Schmidt, S.C., Kakol, J.M., Stein, L.D., Marth, G. *et al.* (2001) A map of human genome sequence variation containing 1.42 million single nucleotide polymorphisms. *Nature*, **409**, 928–933.
3. Thorisson, G.A. and Stein, L.D. (2003) The SNP consortium website: past, present and future. *Nucleic Acids Research*, **31**, 124–127.
4. Brookes, A.J. (1999) The essence of SNPs. *Gene*, **234**, 177–186.
5. Lander, E.S., Linton, L.M., Birren, B., Nusbaum, C., Zody, M.C., Baldwin, J. *et al.* (2001) Initial sequencing and analysis of the human genome. *Nature*, **409**, 860–921.
6. Venter, J.C., Adams, M.D., Myers, E.W., Li, P.W., Mural, R.J., Sutton, G.G. *et al.* (2001) The sequence of the human genome. *Science*, **291**, 1304–1351.
7. Gibbs, R.A., Belmont, J.W., Hardenbol, P., Willis, T.D., Yu, F.L., Yang, H.M. *et al.* (2003) The International HapMap Project. *Nature*, **426**, 789–796.
8. Frazer, K.A., Ballinger, D.G., Cox, D.R., Hinds, D.A., Stuve, L.L., Gibbs, R.A. *et al.* (2007) A second generation human haplotype map of over 3.1 million SNPs. *Nature*, **449**, U851–U853.
9. Musumeci, L., Arthur, J.W., Cheung, F.S.G., Hoque, A., Lippman, S. and Reichardt, J.K.V. (2010) Single Nucleotide Differences (SNDs) in the dbSNP database may lead to errors in genotyping and haplotyping studies. *Human Mutation*, **31**, 67–73.
10. Sherry, S.T., Ward, M.H., Kholodov, M., Baker, J., Phan, L., Smigielski, E.M. *et al.* (2001) dbSNP: the NCBI database of genetic variation. *Nucleic Acids Research*, **29**, 308–311.
11. Ahn, S.M., Kim, T.H., Lee, S., Kim, D., Ghang, H., Kim, D.S. *et al.* (2009) The first Korean genome sequence and analysis: full genome sequencing for a socio-ethnic group. *Genome Research*, **19**, 1622–1629.
12. Bentley, D.R., Balasubramanian, S., Swerdlow, H.P., Smith, G.P., Milton, J., Brown, C.G. *et al.* (2008) Accurate whole human genome sequencing using reversible terminator chemistry. *Nature*, **456**, 53–59.
13. Levy, S., Sutton, G., Ng, P.C., Feuk, L., Halpern, A.L., Walenz, B.P. *et al.* (2007) The diploid genome sequence of an individual human. *PLoS Biology*, **5**, 2113–2144.
14. Schuster, S.C., Miller, W., Ratan, A., Tomsho, L.P., Giardine, B., Kasson, L.R. *et al.* (2010) Complete Khoisan and Bantu genomes from southern Africa. *Nature*, **463**, 943–947.
15. Wang, J., Wang, W., Li, R.Q., Li, Y.R., Tian, G., Goodman, L. *et al.* (2008) The diploid genome sequence of an Asian individual. *Nature*, **456**, U60–U61.
16. Wheeler, D.A., Srinivasan, M., Egholm, M., Shen, Y., Chen, L., McGuire, A. *et al.* (2008) The complete genome of an individual by massively parallel DNA sequencing. *Nature*, **452**, U872–U875.
17. Gill, P. (2001) An assessment of the utility of single nucleotide polymorphisms (SNPs) for forensic purposes. *International Journal of Legal Medicine*, **114**, 204–210.
18. Krawczak, M. (2001) Forensic evaluation of Y-STR haplotype matches: a comment. *Forensic Science International*, **118**, 114–115.
19. Danna, K. and Nathans, D. (1971) Studies of Sv40 DNA. 1. Specific cleavage of Simian virus 40 DNA by restriction endonuclease of Hemophilus influenzae. *Proceedings of the National Academy of Sciences of the United States of America*, **68**, 2913–2291.
20. Denaro, M., Blanc, H., Johnson, M.J., Chen, K.H., Wilmsen, E., Cavallisforza, L.L. *et al.* (1981) Ethnic variation in Hpa-I endonuclease cleavage patterns of human mitochondrial-DNA.

Proceedings of the National Academy of Sciences of the United States of America: Biological Sciences, **78**, 5768–5772.

21. Riehn, R., Lu, M.C., Wang, Y.M., Lim, S.F., Cox, E.C. and Austin, R.H. (2005) Restriction mapping in nanofluidic devices. *Proceedings of the National Academy of Sciences of the United States of America*, **102**, 10012–10016.

22. Sanger, F., Nicklen, S. and Coulson, A.R. (1977) DNA sequencing with chain-terminating inhibitors. *Proceedings of the National Academy of Sciences of the United States of America*, **74**, 5463–5467.

23. Rosenblum, B.B., Lee, L.G., Spurgeon, S.L., Khan, S.H., Menchen, S.M., Heiner, C.R. *et al.* (1997) New dye-labeled terminators for improved DNA sequencing patterns. *Nucleic Acids Research*, **25**, 4500–4504.

24. Prober, J.M., Trainor, G.L., Dam, R.J., Hobbs, F.W., Robertson, C.W., Zagursky, R.J. *et al.* (1987) A system for rapid DNA sequencing with fluorescent chain-terminating dideoxynucleotides. *Science*, **238**, 336–341.

25. Albert, J., Wahlberg, J. and Uhlen, M. (1993) Forensic evidence by DNA sequencing. *Nature*, **361**, 595–596.

26. Metzker, M.L., Mindell, D.P., Liu, X.M., Ptak, R.G., Gibbs, R.A. and Hillis, D.M. (2002) Molecular evidence of HIV-1 transmission in a criminal case. *Proceedings of the National Academy of Sciences of the United States of America*, **99**, 14292–14297.

27. Kwok, P.Y. (2001) Methods for genotyping single nucleotide polymorphisms. *Annual Review of Genomics and Human Genetics*, **2**, 235–258.

28. Syvanen, A.C., Aaltosetala, K., Harju, L., Kontula, K. and Soderlund, H. (1990) A primer-guided nucleotide incorporation assay in the genotyping of apolipoprotein-E. *Genomics*, **8**, 684–692.

29. Sanchez, J.J., Phillips, C., Borsting, C., Balogh, K., Bogus, M., Fondevila, M. *et al.* (2006) A multiplex assay with 52 single nucleotide polymorphisms for human identification. *Electrophoresis*, **27**, 1713–1724.

30. Ronaghi, M., Karamohamed, S., Pettersson, B., Uhlen, M. and Nyren, P. (1996) Real-time DNA sequencing using detection of pyrophosphate release. *Analytical Biochemistry*, **242**, 84–89.

31. Ronaghi, M., Uhlen, M. and Nyren, P. (1998) A sequencing method based on real-time pyrophosphate. *Science*, **281**, 363–336.

32. Fan, J.B., Chen, X.Q., Halushka, M.K., Berno, A., Huang, X.H., Ryder, T. *et al.* (2000) Parallel genotyping of human SNPs using generic high-density oligonucleotide tag arrays. *Genome Research*, **10**, 853–860.

33. Shumaker, J.M., Metspalu, A. and Caskey, C.T. (1996) Mutation detection by solid phase primer extension. *Human Mutation*, **7**, 346–354.

34. Pastinen, T., Raitio, M., Lindroos, K., Tainola, P., Peltonen, L. and Syvanen, A.C. (2000) A system for specific, high-throughput genotyping by allele-specific primer extension on microarrays. *Genome Research*, **10**, 1031–1042.

35. Livak, K.J., Flood, S.J.A., Marmaro, J., Giusti, W. and Deetz, K. (1995) Oligonucleotides with fluorescent dyes at opposite ends provide a quenched probe system useful for detecting PCR product and nucleic-acid hybridization. *PCR-Methods and Applications*, **4**, 357–362.

36. Phillips, C., Fang, R., Ballard, D., Fondevila, M., Harrison, C., Hyland, F. *et al.* (2007) Evaluation of the genplex SNP typing system and a 49 plex forensic marker panel. *Forensic Science International: Genetics*, **1**, 180–185.

37. Saiki, R.K., Bugawan, T.L., Horn, G.T., Mullis, K.B. and Erlich, H.A. (1986) Analysis of enzymatically amplified beta-globin and Hla-Dq-alpha DNA with allele-specific oligonucleotide probes. *Nature*, **324**, 163–166.

38. Lareu, M., Puente, J., Sobrino, B., Quintans, B., Brion, M. and Carracedo, A. (2001) The use of the LightCycler for the detection of Y chromosome SNPs. *Forensic Science International*, **118**, 163–168.

39. Tyagi, S., Bratu, D.P. and Kramer, F.R. (1998) Multicolor molecular beacons for allele discrimination. *Nature Biotechnology*, **16**, 49–53.

40. Tyagi, S. and Kramer, F.R. (1996) Molecular beacons: probes that fluoresce upon hybridization. *Nature Biotechnology*, **14**, 303–308.

41. Wang, D.G., Fan, J.B., Siao, C.J., Berno, A., Young, P., Sapolsky, R. (1998) Large-scale identification, mapping, and genotyping of single-nucleotide polymorphisms in the human genome. *Science*, **280**, 1077–1082.

42. Dixon, L.A., Murray, C.M., Archer, E.J., Dobbins, A.E., Koumi, P. and Gill, P. (2005) Validation of a 21-locus autosomal SNP multiplex for forensic identification purposes. *Forensic Science International*, **154**, 62–77.

43. Inagaki, S., Yamamoto, Y., Doi, Y., Takata, T., Ishikawa, T., Imabayashi, K. *et al.* (2004) A new 39-plex analysis method for SNPs including 15 blood group loci. *Forensic Science International*, **144**, 45–57.

44. Dixon, L.A., Dobbins, A.E., Pulker, H.K., Butler, J.M., Vallone, P.M., Coble, M.D. *et al.* (2006) Analysis of artificially degraded DNA using STRs and SNPs – results of a collaborative European (EDNAP) exercise. *Forensic Science International*, **164**, 33–44.

45. Brion, M., Sanchez, J.J., Balogh, K., Thacker, C., Blanco-Verea, A., Borsting, C. *et al.* (2005) Introduction of an single nucleotide polymorphism-based "Major Y-chromosome haplography typing kit" suitable for predicting the geographical origin of male lineages. *Electrophoresis*, **26**, 4411–4420.

46. Weston, J.H., Tsang, K.W. and Khan, H. (2005) Inferring the population of origin of DNA evidence within the UK by allele-specific hybridization of Y-SNPs. *Forensic Science International*, **152**, 45–53.

47. Freakish, T., Venkateswarlu, K., Thomas, M.J., Gaskin, Z., Ginjupalli, S., Gunturi, S., *et al.* (2003) A classifier for the SNP-based inference of ancestry. *Journal of Forensic Sciences*, **48**, 771–782.

48. Phillips, C., Prieto, L., Fondevila, M., Salas, A., Gomez-Tato, A., Alvarez-Dios, J. *et al.* (2009) Ancestry analysis in the 11-M Madrid bomb attack investigation. *PLoS One*, **4**, e6583.

49. Bastiaens, M., ter Huurne, J., Gruis, N., Bergman, W., Westendorp, R., Vermeer, B.J. *et al.* (2001) The melanocortin-1-receptor gene is the major freckle gene. *Human Molecular Genetics*, **10**, 1701–1708.

50. Duffy, D.L., Montgomery, G.W., Chen, W., Zhao, Z.Z., Le, L., James, M.R. *et al.* (2007) A three–single-nucleotide polymorphism haplotype in intron 1 of OCA2 explains most human eye-color variation. *American Journal of Human Genetics*, **80**, 241–252.

51. Grimes, E.A., Noake, P.J., Dixon, L. and Urquhart, A. (2001) Sequence polymorphism in the human melanocortin 1 receptor gene as an indicator of the red hair phenotype. *Forensic Science International*, **122**, 124–129.

52. Sturm, R.A., Zhao, Z.Z., Leite, F.P.N., Stark, M.S., Hayward, N.K. *et al.* (2008) A single SNP in an evolutionary conserved region within intron 86 of the HERC2 gene determines human blue-brown eye color. *American Journal of Human Genetics*, **82**, 424–431.

53. Doi, Y., Yamamoto, Y., Inagaki, S., Shigeta, Y., Miyaishi, S., Ishizu, H. (2004) A new method for ABO genotyping using a multiplex single-base primer extension reaction and its application to forensic casework samples. *Legal Medicine*, **6**, 213–223.

54. Ackerman, M.J., Tester, D.J., Driscoll, D.J. (2001) Molecular autopsy of sudden unexplained death in the young. *American Journal of Forensic Medicine and Pathology*, **22**, 105–111.

55. Levo, A., Koski, A., Ojanpera, I., Vuori, E. and Sajantila, A. (2003) Post-mortem SNP analysis of CYP2D6 gene reveals correlation between genotype and opioid drug (tramadol) metabolite ratios in blood. *Forensic Science International*, **135**, 9–15.

13 Lineage markers

Genetic lineage markers comprise polymorphisms that are present on the maternally inherited mitochondrial genome and the paternally inherited Y chromosome. The analysis of lineage markers is limited in most forensic casework because they do not possess the power of discrimination of autosomal markers. Even so, there are some features of both mtDNA and the Y chromosome that make them valuable forensic tools.

Mitochondria

The mitochondria are organelles that exist in the cytoplasm of eukaryotic cells. They carry out the vital job of producing approximately 90% of the energy required by the cell through the process of oxidative phosphorylation.

Inheritance of the mitochondrial genome

Mitochondria contain their own genome (mtDNA), which is maternally inherited [1, 2]. This was discovered in the 1950s after unusual patterns of inheritance of certain phenotypes were explained by the existence of extra-nuclear genomes that did not obey Mendel's laws of inheritance.

During fertilization of an ovum, the sperm penetrates the ovum and the sperm mid-piece, which contains between 50 and 75 mitochondria, enters the ovum along with the head [3]. The ovum has around 1000 times more mitochondria than the sperm [3]. Although some paternal mtDNA enters the ovum it is actively removed [4]. The process is not always completely effective and very rare cases of paternal mtDNA inheritance have been documented [5].

Copy number

The mtDNA genome is present in multiple copies: individual cells can contain hundreds of mitochondria and a single human mitochondrion can contain several copies of the genome [6–8]. Somatic cells, therefore, have thousands of copies of the mitochondrial genome and approximately 1% of total cellular DNA comprises mtDNA [9, 10]. This compares with only two copies per cell of the nuclear genome.

The mtDNA genome

The human mitochondrial genome is a 16 569 bp circular molecule. It encodes for 22 transfer RNAs (tRNAs), 13 proteins and two ribosomal RNAs (the 12S and 16S rRNAs) [11, 12]. The majority of mitochondrial proteins is encoded by the nuclear genome as, over hundreds of millions of years, following the formation of the symbiotic relationship between eubacteria and eukaryote cells, most of the genes have been transferred from the mitochondrial to the nuclear genome [13]. Analysis of the human mtDNA genome revealed a very economic use of the DNA and there are very few non-coding bases within the genome except in a region called the D-loop (Figure 13.1). The D-loop is the region of the genome where the initial separation, or displacement, of the two strands of DNA during replication occurs. The regulatory role of the D-loop has led to the other name by which it is known – the control region. It is approximately 1100 bp long.

Polymorphisms in mtDNA

The mtDNA genome accumulates mutations relatively rapidly when compared with the nuclear genome [14]. The high mutation rate[1] is due in part to the exposure of the

Figure 13.1   The mitochondrial genome is circular and 16 569 bp long. It encodes for 13 proteins 22 transfer RNAs and two ribosomal RNAs. The polymorphic hypervariable regions I and II (HV-I, HV-II and HV-III) are located within the control region. Other regions of the genome that are utilized in forensic casework for species identification are the coding regions for the 12S and 16S ribosomal RNAs, cytochrome *c* oxidase subunit I (COI) gene and cytochrome *b* gene

---

[1] Note: Mutations in the hypervariable regions are normally referred to as 'a base substitution' as they do not have an effect on any of the products encoded by the mtDNA – for simplicity the term 'mutation' will be used throughout this chapter.

mtDNA to reactive oxygen species that are produced as byproducts in oxidative phosphorylation [15]. Direct analysis of mother-to-children transmissions has estimated that a mutation in the hypervariable regions is passed from mother to child approximately once in every 30–40 events. In the vast majority of cases where a mutation is detected, there is only one base change between the mother and child [16, 17].

Hypervariable regions

In most forensic investigations the aim of DNA profiling is to differentiate between individuals; therefore, the most polymorphic regions are analysed. Following the sequencing of the human mtDNA genome it was apparent that the D-loop, also known as the control region, was not under the same functional constraints as the rest of the genome. Some blocks within the control region are highly conserved but large parts are not. Two main regions are the focus of most forensic studies, these are known as hypervariable sequence regions I and II (HV-I and HV-II) and they contain the highest levels of variation within the mtDNA genome. Both the hypervariable blocks are approximately 350 bp long. A third hypervariable region, HV-III has also been used in some cases. Within the hypervariable regions the rate of mutation is not constant and some sites are hotspots for mutation, whereas others show much lower rates of change [18–20].

The polymorphic sites are concentrated within relatively small regions of the mtDNA genome and can be analysed using PCR amplification followed by Sanger sequencing [21]. Many of the methods used for SNP detection can also be used (see Chapter 12).

Applications of mtDNA profiling

There are several scenarios where mtDNA is a valuable genetic marker. These are related to two properties of mtDNA – the high copy number and the maternal inheritance. The high copy number is valuable when the amount of cellular material available for analysis is very small: crime scene material that is commonly profiled using mtDNA includes hair shafts [22–24] and faecal samples [25].

mtDNA is also useful for the analysis of human remains that are highly degraded and not amenable to standard STR typing [26–29]. The maternal inheritance is a useful trait for human identification when there are no direct relatives to use as a reference sample; the identification of some of the Romanov family using Prince Philip and other living relatives as reference samples provides a powerful illustration of the use of maternal inheritance [30, 31] (Figure 13.2).

A series of historical cases has followed that demonstrates the application of mtDNA when linking relatives to human remains [32–37].

Interpretation of mtDNA profiles

mtDNA is used for both associating crime scene samples with individuals and also in the identification of human remains. In both cases the profile that has been generated

Figure 13.2 The family tree of the Romanov royal family: (a) shows the maternal lineage of the Tsarina and her children which provides a direct link to Prince Philip and (b) illustrates the maternal lineage of Tsar Nicholas, linking him to two living maternal relatives, the Duke of Fife and Xenia Cheremeteff-Sfiri. The squares represent males and the circles represent females, the transmission of the relevant mtDNA type is in red

from the unknown sample has to be compared with a reference profile. In the case of a crime scene investigation, the reference sample will be from a suspect. In the case of human identification, a sample taken from a maternal relative or a personal artefact such as a toothbrush can be used [38].

The first step is to turn the information into a more manageable form. The data after sequencing consist of upwards of 350 DNA bases from both HV-I and HV-II and around 150 bases from HV-III. Once the sequencing data have been checked to ensure that there is confidence in the sequence data and no errors, it is compared with the Cambridge Reference Sequence (CRS) [11, 12]. The CRS was the first complete sequence of the mtDNA genome to be published in 1981. Differences between the questioned sequence and the CRS are noted and only these differences are recorded. Table 13.1 shows an example of where a HV-I profile generated from a set of human remains is compared with profiles generated from three reference samples. The mtDNA profile is called a haplotype.

Homoplasmy and heteroplasmy

Normally an individual contains only one type of mtDNA: this is termed homoplasmy (Figure 13.3). Mutations will inevitably occur within some of the thousands of copies of mtDNA within a cell and if these mutated copies of the genome were passed on to future generations, a mixture of different mtDNA genomes would occur. The process that maintains homoplasmy as the norm is not precisely understood but at some point a genetic bottleneck occurs before the formation of a mature oocyte [40]. The bottleneck allows only a few mtDNA molecules to pass into the oocyte during its formation [41, 42], thereby reducing the possibility of passing on a mixture of wild type and mutant genomes.

Table 13.1 An example where an mtDNA profile has been generated from the HV-I of five bones that were found in close proximity. The mtDNA profiles of three women who were maternal relatives of three missing individuals are also shown. Maternal reference 1 clearly matches the bone, while maternal reference 2 and 3 can be excluded as potential maternal relatives as they have different mtDNA types. In this particular case the mtDNA profiling helped to establish the identification of the human remains, and that the bones all came from the same person [39]

Sample	HV-I sequence			
Right femur	16 189C	16 223T	16 271C	16 278T
Left femur	16 189C	16 223T	16 271C	16 278T
Right pelvis	16 189C	16 223T	16 271C	16 278T
Left ulna	16 189C	16 223T	16 271C	16 278T
Left tibia	16 189C	16 223T	16 271C	16 278T
Maternal reference 1	16 189C	16 223T	16 271C	16 278T
Maternal reference 2	Same as Cambridge Reference Sequence			
Maternal reference 3	16 278T	16 293G	16 311C	–

Figure 13.3 The above sequence shows the presence of heteroplasmy at position 16 189, two bases, a C and an A, are present in approximately equal amounts

It is, however, possible to find more than one type of mtDNA within a cell: this is known as heteroplasmy and it arises when a mother passes on a normal version of her mtDNA genome (wild type) and also a version of the genome that contains a mutation. An individual will therefore possess two versions of mtDNA, usually only differing by one base [22, 23] but have been observed to differ at two and even three positions [43]. Two factors, the severity of the bottleneck and subsequent genetic drift, determine the relative levels of wild to mutated mtDNA [16, 17]. Heteroplasmy can be stable through several generations before one of the mtDNA versions becomes fixed [16, 17, 32, 41, 44].

Haplotypes and haplogroups

The sequence of a particular mtDNA genome is its haplotype (see Table 13.1). mtDNA genomes that are not identical, but closely related are said to be within the same haplogroup: mtDNA can be assigned to a haplogroup based on containing characteristic mutations; some of these are within the hypervariable region, whereas others are dispersed around the genome; the evolutionary relationship of different haplogroups can be shown as a phylogenetic tree [45, 46]. mtDNA haplogroups show geographical clustering, so, for example haplogroup H occurs at a frequency of approximately 40% in western Europeans, whereas it is virtually absent from Africa and Southeast Asia. Based on the relative frequency of the haplogroups in different geographic populations, the geographical origin of a particular sample can therefore be inferred [47–49]. In a forensic investigation care should be taken not to overinterpret the 'ethnicity' prediction of a sample left at a crime scene as it only shows the maternal lineage, which may have become admixed with another geographic population several generations ago.

Evaluation of mtDNA profiles

Declaring a match is straightforward, but exclusions can be more problematic. When a questioned sample and a reference sample differ at only one position the likelihood of that one base difference occurring though a mutation has to be assessed. In such an instance the results are usually classified as inconclusive – when there are two or more differences between a questioned and known sample it is normally classified as an exclusion [21].

If a match is declared, the statistical significance has to be assessed. The mtDNA genome is inherited as a single locus and this limits the evidential value in forensic cases. Haplotype frequencies have to be measured directly by counting the occurrence of a particular haplotype in a database and reporting the size of the database [50]. When databases are relatively small, for example 100, many of the less common haplotypes that are within a population will not be represented. There are mechanisms that compensate for the limitations of reference databases, such as minimum haplotype frequencies, employing standard error calculations and correction factors to allow for subpopulations [51, 52].

If a mtDNA haplotype occurs at a relatively high frequency in the population of interest then additional information can be gained by typing some of the polymorphisms that occur outside the hypervariable regions, thereby increasing the evidential value of the mtDNA [53–55].

When reporting the results of mtDNA analysis, the caveats associated with mtDNA have to be clearly explained so that there is no confusion with 'standard' (autosomal STR typing) analysis. In particular that 'it is inherited only from one's mother, and therefore all individuals who are related by a maternal link will have the same mtDNA profile', and that 'it varies less between individuals, and therefore more individuals chosen at random from the population will have the same mtDNA profile' should be made very clear.

The Y chromosome

In humans the Y chromosome is approximately 60 Mb long (million base pairs) long and contains just 78 genes [56]. The SRY gene (sex-determining region Y) located on the Y chromosome encodes a protein that triggers the development of the testes and through an extended hormonal pathway causes a developing fetus to become male [57].

With the exception of two regions, PAR 1 and 2 (PAR = pseudoautosomal region), located at the tips of the chromosome, no recombination occurs during meiosis. The remaining 95% of the Y chromosome is non-recombining, male specific and is passed from father to son unchanged, except when mutations occur. The lack of recombination may be the reason why there are relatively few genes on the Y chromosome. If there is no chromosome crossing-over, mutations within genes have little chance to be repaired or rectified and hence will be passed on to the next generation.

Y chromosome polymorphisms

The Y chromosome contains a large number of polymorphisms including VNTRs [58] and STRs, insertions, deletions and SNPs. As with mtDNA, the polymorphisms can be used to classify Y chromosomes into a series of haplogroups; SNPs that have occurred only once in the evolution of the Y chromosome are used for haplogroup designation [59].

Most forensic work utilizes haplotypes based on STRs. The first STR locus to be identified on the Y chromosome was DYS19 [60]. Since then hundreds of Y chromosome STRs have been described. The development of Y STR typing has mirrored the development of the autosomal STRs, and multiplexes have been developed with increasing numbers of robust and highly discriminating Y STR multiplexes [61–64]. The growth in interest in Y STR loci has led to numerous population studies to establish allele frequency databases. The Y Chromosome Haplotype Reference Database (yhrd) was established to collate STR haplotypes (www.yhrd.org). To ensure comparability between datasets, minimal and extended haplotypes were defined. Two commercial kits, the PowerPlex® Y (Promega Corporation) and the AmpFℓSTR® Yfiler® (Applied Biosystems) incorporate all of the extended haplotype loci (Table 13.2).

The techniques used for profiling are the same as for autosomal STRs (see Chapter 6). The only notable difference is that a Y chromosome profile, with the exception of DYS385 a/b and DYS389 I, contains one allele at each locus (Figure 13.4). The locus DYS385 is duplicated on the Y chromosome and the PCR primers recognize both copies of the locus; the DYS389 locus is complex with two polymorphic regions, the PCR primers amplify DYS389I, which is a polymorphic element within the locus and DYS389II is the whole locus.

Table 13.2 The Y chromosome STR loci that are commonly used in forensic analysis

Minimal haplotype	Extended haplotype	PowerPlex® Y	AmpFℓSTR® Yfiler®
DYS19	DYS19	DYS19	DYS19
DYS385 a/b	DYS385 a/b	DYS385 a/b	DYS385 a/b
DYS389 I	DYS389 I	DYS389 I	DYS389 I
DYS389 II	DYS389 II	DYS389 II	DYS389 II
DYS390	DYS390	DYS390	DYS390
DYS391	DYS391	DYS391	DYS391
DYS392	DYS392	DYS392	DYS392
DYS393	DYS393	DYS393	DYS393
	DYS438	DYS437	DYS437
	DYS439	DYS438	DYS438
		DYS439	DYS439
			DYS448
			DYS456
			DYS458
			DYS635
			GATA H4

The Y chromosome is effectively digitized, and based on the example in Figure 13.4 can be represented as a series of 17 numbers, making comparisons and database searching relatively simple. The result of a search of the yhrd is shown in Figure 13.5.

Forensic applications of Y chromosome polymorphisms

That the Y chromosome is only found in males makes it a valuable tool, in particular for the analysis of male and female mixtures after sexual assaults when differential DNA extraction is not possible; Y STR analysis has been successful with female–male ratios of up to 2000:1 [65]. The presence of male DNA has also been detected when vaginal swabs were analysed, even when no spermatozoa have been detected – either through the assailant being azoospermic (1–2% of rape cases) or through the deterioration of the spermatozoa [62, 66]. The Y STRs can also be used to detect the presence of two male profiles; the interpretation of the mixtures depends on the presence of major and minor contributors [65].

Y chromosome profiling has also been used for paternity testing and is particularly valuable in deficient cases, where the alleged father is not available for testing. In these cases, any male relative who is paternally related to the alleged father can be used as a reference. An extreme example of where this has been used is the paternity analysis that linked the third US president, Thomas Jefferson, to the child of one of his slaves, Sally Hemings [67, 68]. Cases involving human identification have also used the Y chromosome as a tool to link remains to paternal family members, and as with deficient paternity cases the use of the Y chromosome is particularly advantageous when there are no parents or children to use as reference material; it also simplifies the sorting of the material following mass disasters [69].

Figure 13.4 Profile of a Y chromosome using the AmpFℓSTR® YFiler®, which amplifies 16 STR loci. The allelic designation is shown at each locus along with the size of the amplified PCR product

Figure 13.5 The Y chromosome profile shown in Figure 13.4 was searched against the YSTR database (http://www.yhrd.org). In this case the haplotype had not been seen before in any of the 26 136 samples present in the database

The Y chromosome has a non-random distribution among global populations, largely due to the widespread practice of patrilocality [70, 71] (where the female moves to the male's birth place/residence after marriage). This makes it a useful tool for inferring the geographical origins of biological material recovered from a crime scene and human remains [72]. As with mtDNA, the inferences regarding geographical origins have to be treated with caution. Finally, in cultures where the male name is passed on to male children, there is also the potential, of attributing surnames to Y profiles, which has the potential to be useful [73, 74].

Evaluation of Y STR profiles

When the Y chromosome profiles from a reference and an unknown sample match, the significance of the match has to be assessed. The first step is to assess the frequencies of the Y STR haplotypes in the population of interest. The simplest method is to report the frequency of the Y STR haplotype in the population, known as the counting method. The figure quoted is entirely dependent upon the size of the database and is normally based on frequency databases that are constructed for the major ethnic groups represented within individual countries, although comparisons can also be made with the combined data in the yhrd databases with over 80 000 haplotypes (representing at least the minimal haplotype). So, for example a match can be reported as 'the haplotype has been seen twice in 400 UK Caucasian individuals'. Corrections can be made to allow for sampling error in the reference databases [75, 76].

The Y chromosome will accumulate mutations as it is passed through the patrilineal line and direct comparison between males on the same lineage may result in a false exclusion if mutations are not considered. The mutation rate in Y STR loci is similar to autosomal STRs, at approximately 2.8×10^{-3} [75, 77–79]. Although most mutation events affect only one locus, there is at least one observed instance where three Y chromosome STRs differed between a father and son [80].

Further difficulties arise in the interpretation of the Y chromosome because of the patrilineal inheritance and clustering of male family members in relatively small geographic areas. This geographical clustering of male relatives coupled with the limited size of the haplotype frequency databases (many haplotypes are seen only once) makes the estimation of profile frequencies hazardous [81]. An alternative method for assessing the significance of a match is to use a likelihood ratio and to incorporate population subdivisions with the increased potential for common co-ancestry [52]. Regardless of the method used to calculate the matching frequency, when presenting the results of Y chromosome analysis, as with mtDNA, there is a need to state how the use of Y STR typing varies from that of autosomal markers and that there will be other males in the population with the same Y STR haplotype.

Further reading

Jobling, M., Hurles, M. and Tyler-Smith, C. (2004) *Human Evolutionary Genetics: Origins, Peoples and Disease*, Garland Science.
Cavalli-Sforza, L.L., Menozzi, P. and Piazza, A. (1996) *The History and Geography of Human Genes*, Princeton University Press.

WWW resources

The Y Chromosome Haplotype Reference Database. http://www.yhrd.org.
EMPOP – Mitochondrial DNA Control Region Database. http://www.empop.org/.
MITOMAP. http://www.mitomap.org/.

References

1. Giles, R.E., Blanc, H., Cann, H.M. and Wallace, D.C. (1980) Maternal inheritance of human mitochondrial-DNA. *Proceedings of the National Academy of Sciences of the United States of America-Biological Sciences*, **77**, 6715–6719.
2. Shitara, H., Hayashi, J., Takahama, S., Kaneda, H. and Yonekawa, H. (1998) Maternal inheritance of mouse mtDNA in interspecific hybrids: segregation of the leaked paternal mtDNA followed by the prevention of subsequent paternal leakage. *Genetics*, **148**, 851–857.
3. Ankel-Simons, F. and Cummins, J.M. (1996) Misconceptions about mitochondria and mammalian fertilization: Implications for theories on human evolution. *Proceedings of the National Academy of Sciences of the United States of America*, **93**, 13859–13863.
4. Thompson, W.E., Ramalho-Santos, J. and Sutovsky, P. (2003) Ubiquitination of prohibitin in mammalian sperm mitochondria: Possible roles in the regulation of mitochondrial inheritance and sperm quality control. *Biology of Reproduction*, **69**, 254–260.
5. Schwartz, M. and Vissing, J. (2002) Paternal inheritance of mitochondrial DNA. *New England Journal of Medicine*, **347**, 576–580.
6. Cavelier, L., Johannisson, A. and Gyllensten, U. (2000) Analysis of mtDNA copy number and composition of single mitochondrial particles using flow cytometry and PCR. *Experimental Cell Research*, **259**, 79–85.
7. Garrido, N., Griparic, L., Jokitalo, E., Wartiovaara, J., van der Bliek, A.M. and Spelbrink, J.N. (2003) Composition and dynamics of human mitochondrial nucleoids. *Molecular Biology of the Cell*, **14**, 1583–1596.
8. Margineantu, D.H., Cox, W.G., Sundell, L., Sherwood, S.W., Beechem, J.A. and Capaldi, R.A. (2002) Cell cycle dependent morphology changes and associated mitochondrial DNA redistribution in mitochondria of human cell lines. *Mitochondrion*, **1**, 425–435.
9. Bogenhag, D. and Clayton, D.A. (1974) Number of mitochondrial deoxyribonucleic-acid genomes in mouse L and human Hela-cells – quantitative isolation of mitochondrial deoxyribonucleic-acid. *Journal of Biological Chemistry*, **249**, 7991–7995.
10. Robin, E.D. and Wong, R. (1988) Mitochondrial-DNA molecules and virtual number of mitochondria per cell in mammalian-cells. *Journal of Cellular Physiology*, **136**, 507–513.
11. Anderson, S., Bankier, A.T., Barrell, B.G., Debruijn, M.H.L., Coulson, A.R. and Drouin, J. (1981)· Sequence and organization of the human mitochondrial genome. *Nature*, **290**, 457–465.
12. Andrews, R.M., Kubacka, I., Chinnery, P.F., Lightowlers, R.N., Turnbull, D.M. and Howell, N. (1999) Reanalysis and revision of the Cambridge reference sequence for human mitochondrial DNA. *Nature Genetics*, **23**, 147–147.

13. Dyall, S.D., Brown, M.T. and Johnson, P.J. (2004) Ancient invasions: from endosymbionts to organelles. *Science*, **304**, 253–257.
14. Brown, W.M., George, M. and Wilson, A.C. (1979) Rapid evolution of animal mitochondrial-DNA. *Proceedings of the National Academy of Sciences of the United States of America*, **76**, 1967–1971.
15. Hashiguchi, K., Bohr, VA, de Souza-Pinto, NC. (2004) Oxidative stress and mitochondrial DNA repair: implications for NRTIs induced DNA damage. *Mitochondrion*, **4**, 215–222.
16. Forster, L., Forster, P., Lutz-Bonengel, S., Willkomm, H. and Brinkmann, B. (2002) Natural radioactivity and human mitochondrial DNA mutations. *Proceedings of the National Academy of Sciences of the United States of America*, **99**, 13950–13954.
17. Parsons, T.J., Muniec, D.S., Sullivan, K., Woodyatt, N., AllistonGreiner, R., Wilson, M.R. *et al.* (1997) A high observed substitution rate in the human mitochondrial DNA control region. *Nature Genetics*, **15**, 363–368.
18. Excoffier, L. and Yang, Z.H. (1999) Substitution rate variation among sites in mitochondrial hypervariable region I of humans and chimpanzees. *Molecular Biology and Evolution*, **16**, 1357–1368.
19. Meyer, S., Weiss, G. and von Haeseler, A. (1999) Pattern of nucleotide substitution and rate heterogeneity in the hypervariable regions I and II of human mtDNA. *Genetics*, **152**, 1103–1110.
20. Tamura, K. and Nei, M. (1993) Estimation of the number of nucleotide substitutions in the control region of mitochondrial-DNA in humans and chimpanzees. *Molecular Biology and Evolution*, **10**, 512–526.
21. Carracedo, A., Bar, W., Lincoln, P., Mayr, W., Morling, N. and Olaisen, B. *et al.* (2000) DNA commission of the international society for forensic genetics: guidelines for mitochondrial DNA typing. *Forensic Science International*, **110**, 79–85.
22. Melton, T., Dimick, G., Higgins, B., Lindstrom, L. and Nelson, K. (2005) Forensic mitochondrial DNA analysis of 691 casework hairs. *Journal of Forensic Sciences*, **50**, 73–80.
23. Melton, T. and Nelson, K. (2001) Forensic mitochondrial DNA analysis: two years of commercial casework experience in the United States. *Croatian Medical Journal*, **42**, 298–202.
24. Szibor, R. Plate I, Schmitter H, Wittig H, Krause D. (2006) Forensic mass screening using mtDNA. *International Journal of Legal Medicine*, **120**, 372–376.
25. Hopwood, A.J., Mannucci, A. and Sullivan, K.M. (1996) DNA typing from human faeces. *International Journal of Legal Medicine*, **108**, 237–243.
26. Goodwin, W., Linacre, A. and Vanezis, P. (1999) The use of mitochondrial DNA and short tandem repeat typing in the identification of air crash victims. *Electrophoresis*, **20**, 1707–1711.
27. Holland, M.M., Fisher, D.L., Mitchell, L.G., Rodriguez, W.C., Canik, J.J. and Merril, C.R. (1993) Mitochondrial-DNA sequence-analysis of human skeletal remains – identification of remains from the Vietnam-War. *Journal of Forensic Sciences*, **38**, 542–553.
28. Sudoyo, H., Widodo, P.T., Suryadi, H., Lie, Y.S., Safari, D. and Widjajanto, A. (2008) DNA analysis in perpetrator identification of terrorism-related disaster: suicide bombing of the Australian Embassy in Jakarta 2004. *Forensic Science International: Genetics*, **2**, 231–237.
29. Nelson, K. and Melton, T. (2007) Forensic mitochondrial DNA analysis of 116 casework skeletal samples. *Journal of Forensic Sciences*, **52**, 557–561.
30. Gill, P., Ivanov, P.L., Kimpton, C., Piercy, R., Benson, N. and Tully, G. (1994) Identification of the remains of the Romanov family by DNA analysis. *Nature Genetics*, **6**, 130–135.
31. Coble, M.D., Loreille, O.M., Wadhams, M.J., Edson, S.M., Maynard, K. and Meyer, C.E. (2009) Mystery solved: the identification of the two missing Romanov children using DNA analysis. *PLoS One*, **4**, e4838.
32. Ivanov, P.L., Wadhams, M.J., Roby, R.K., Holland, M.M., Weedn, V.W. and Parsons, T.J. (1996) Mitochondrial DNA sequence heteroplasmy in the Grand Duke of Russia Georgij Romanov establishes the authenticity of the remains of TsarNicholas II. *Nature Genetics*, **12**, 417–420.
33. Stoneking, M., Melton, T., Nott, J., Barritt, S., Roby, R. and Holland, M. (1995) Establishing the identity of Anna Manahan Anderson. *Nature Genetics*, **9**, 9–10.

34. Stone, A.C., Starrs, J.E. and Stoneking, M. (2001) Mitochondrial DNA analysis of the presumptive remains of Jesse James. *Journal of Forensic Sciences*, **46**, 173–176.

35. Bogdanowicz, W., Allen, M., Branicki, W., Lembring, M., Gajewska, M. and Kupiec, T. (2009) Genetic identification of putative remains of the famous astronomer Nicolaus Copernicus. *Proceedings of the National Academy of Sciences of the United States of America*, **106**, 12279–12282.

36. Gilbert, M.T.R., Djurhuus, D., Melchior, L., Lynnerup, N., Worobey, M., Wilson, A.S. *et al.* (2007) mtDNA from hair and nail clarifies the genetic relationship of the 15th century Qilakitsoq Inuit mummies. *American Journal of Physical Anthropology*, **133**, 847–853.

37. Dissing, J., Binladen, J., Hansen, A., Sejrsen, B., Willerslev, E. and Lynnerup, N. (2007) The last Viking King: a royal maternity case solved by ancient DNA analysis. *Forensic Science International*, **166**, 21–27.

38. Brenner, C.H. and Weir, B.S. (2003) Issues and strategies in the DNA identification of World Trade Center victims. *Theoretical Population Biology*, **63**, 173–178.

39. Goodwin, W., McFarlane, J. and Roberts, J. (2003) The identification of a US serviceman recovered from the Holy Loch, Scotland. *Science and Justice*, **43**, 45–47.

40. Marchington, D.R., Macaulay, V., Hartshorne, G.M., Barlow, D. and Poulton, J. (1998) Evidence from human oocytes for a genetic bottleneck in an mtDNA disease. *American Journal of Human Genetics*, **63**, 769–775.

41. Chinnery, P.F., Thorburn, D.R., Samuels, D.C., White, S.L., Dahl, H.H.M. and Turnbull, D.M. (2000) The inheritance of mitochondrial DNA heteroplasmy: random drift, selection or both? *Trends in Genetics*, **16**, 500–505.

42. Sekiguchi, K., Kasai, K. and Levin, B.C. (2003) Inter- and intragenerational transmission of a human mitochondrial DNA heteroplasmy among 13 maternally-related individuals and differences between and within tissues in two family members. *Mitochondrion*, **2**, 401–414.

43. Irwin, J.A., Saunier, J.L., Niederstatter, H., Strouss, K.M., Sturk, K.A. and Diegoli, T.M. (2009) Investigation of heteroplasmy in the human mitochondrial DNA control region: a synthesis of observations from more than 5000 global population samples. *Journal of Molecular Evolution*, **68**, 516–527.

44. Lagerstrom-Fermer, M., Olsson, C., Forsgren, L. and Syvanen, A.C. (2001) Heteroplasmy of the human mtDNA control region remains constant during life. *American Journal of Human Genetics*, **68**, 1299–1301.

45. van Oven, M. and Kayser, M. (2009) Updated comprehensive phylogenetic tree of global human mitochondrial DNA variation. *Human Mutation*, **30**, E386–E394.

46. Salas, A., Bandelt, H.J., Macaulay, V. and Richards, M.B. (2007) Phylogeographic investigations: the role of trees in forensic genetics. *Forensic Science International*, **168**, 1–13.

47. Tokutomi, T., Takada, Y., Murayama, T., Mukaida, M. and Kanetake, J. (2009) Real-time PCR method for identification of Asian populations in forensic casework. *Legal Medicine (Tokyo)*, **11** (Suppl 1), S106–S108.

48. Phillips, C., Prieto, L., Fondevila, M., Salas, A., Gomez-Tato, A. and Alvarez-Dios, J. (2009) Ancestry analysis in the 11-M Madrid bomb attack investigation. *PLoS One*, **4**, e6583.

49. Parson, W., Fendt, L., Ballard, D., Borsting, C., Brinkmann, B. and Carracedo, A. (2008) Identification of West Eurasian mitochondrial haplogroups by mtDNA SNP screening: results of the 2006–2007 EDNAP collaborative exercise. *Forensic Science International: Genetics*, **2**, 61–68.

50. Parson, W. and Dur, A. (2007) EMPOP – a forensic mtDNA database. *Forensic Science International: Genetics*, **1**, 88–92.

51. Balding, D.J. and Nichols, R.A. (1994) DNA profile match probability calculation – how to allow for population stratification, relatedness, database selection and single bands. *Forensic Science International*, **64**, 125–140.

52. Buckleton, J., Triggs, C.M. and Walsh, S.J. (2005) *Forensic DNA Evidence Interpretation*, CRC Press.

53. Irwin, J.A., Edson, S.M., Loreille, O., Just, R.S., Barritt, S.M., Lee, D.A. *et al.* (2007) DNA identification of "Earthquake McGoon" 50 years postmortem. *Journal of Forensic Sciences*, **52**, 1115–1118.

54. Just, R.S., Irwin, J.A., O'Callaghan, J.E., Saunier, J.L., Coble, M.D., Vallone, P.M. *et al.* (2004) Toward increased utility of mtDNA in forensic identifications. *Forensic Sciences International*, **146**, S147–S149.

55. Coble, M.D., Just, R.S., O'Callaghan, J.E., Letmanyi, I.H., Peterson, C.T., Irwin, J.A. *et al.* (2004) Single nucleotide polymorphisms over the entire mtDNA genome that increase the power of forensic testing in Caucasians. *International Journal of Legal Medicine*, **118**, 137–146.

56. Skaletsky, H., Kuroda-Kawaguchi, T., Minx, P.J., Cordum, H.S., Hillier, L., Brown, L.G. *et al.* (2003) The male-specific region of the human Y chromosome is a mosaic of discrete sequence classes. *Nature*, **423**, U825–U822.

57. Sinclair, A.H., Berta, P., Palmer, M.S., Hawkins, J.R., Griffiths, B.L., Smith, M.J. *et al.* (1990) A gene from the human sex-determining region encodes a protein with homology to a conserved DNA-binding motif. *Nature*, **346**, 240–244.

58. Jobling, M.A., Bouzekri, N. and Taylor, P.G. (1998) Hypervariable digital DNA codes for human paternal lineages: MVR-PCR at the Y-specific minisatellite, MSY1 (DYF155S1). *Human Molecular Genetics*, **7**, 643–653.

59. Shi, W.T., Ayub, Q., Vermeulen, M., Shao, R.G., Zuniga, S., van der Gaag, K. *et al.* (2010) A worldwide survey of human male demographic history based on Y-SNP and Y-STR data from the HGDP-CEPH populations. *Molecular Biology and Evolution*, **27**, 385–393.

60. Roewer, L., Arnemann, J., Spurr, N.K., Grzeschik, K.H. and Epplen, J.T. (1992) Simple repeat sequences on the human Y-chromosome are equally polymorphic as their autosomal counterparts. *Human Genetics*, **89**, 389–394.

61. Butler, J.M., Schoske, R., Vallone, P.M., Kline, M.C., Redd, A.J. and Hammer, M.F. (2002) A novel multiplex for simultaneous amplification of 20 Y chromosome STR markers. *Forensic Science International*, **129**, 10–24.

62. Gusmao, L., Brion, M., Gonzalez-Neira, A., Lareu, M. and Carracedo, A. (1999) Y chromosome specific polymorphisms in forensic analysis. *Legal Medicine*, **1**, 55–60.

63. Mulero, J.J., Chang, C.W., Calandro, L.M., Green, R.L., Li, Y., and Johnson, C.L. (2006) Development and validation of the AmpFlSTR (R) Yfiler (TM) PCR amplification kit: a male specific, single amplification 17 Y-STR multiplex system. *Journal of Forensic Sciences*, **51**, 64–75.

64. Krenke, B.E., Viculis, L., Richard, M.L., Prinz, M., Milne, S.C., Ladd, C. *et al.* (2005) Validation of a male-specific, 12-locus fluorescent short tandem repeat (STR) multiplex. *Forensic Science International*, **148**, 1–14.

65. Prinz, M., Boll, K., Baum, H. and Shaler, B. (1997) Multiplexing of Y chromosome specific STRs and performance for mixed samples. *Forensic Science International*, **85**, 209–218.

66. Sibille, I., Duverneuil, C., de la Grandmaison, G.L., Guerrouache, K., Teissiere, F., Durigon, M. *et al.* (2002) Y-STR DNA amplification as biological evidence in sexually assaulted female victims with no cytological detection of spermatozoa. *Forensic Science International*, **125**, 212–216.

67. Foster, E.A., Jobling, M.A., Taylor, P.G., Donnelly, P., de Knijff, P., Mieremet, R. *et al.* (1998) Jefferson fathered slave's last child. *Nature*, **396**, 27–28.

68. Foster, E.A., Jobling, M.A., Taylor, P.G., Donnelly, P., de Knijff, P., Mieremet, R. *et al.* (1999) The Thomas Jefferson paternity case – Reply. *Nature*, **397**, 32–32.

69. Corach, D., Risso, L.F., Marino, M., Penacino, G. and Sala, A. (2001) Routine Y-STR typing in forensic casework. *Forensic Science International*, **118**, 131–135.

70. Burton, M.L., Moore, C.C., Whiting, J.W.M. and Romney, A.K. (1996) Regions based on social structure. *Current Anthropology*, **37**, 87–123.

71. Oota, H., Settheetham-Ishida, W., Tiwawech, D., Ishida, T. and Stoneking, M. (2001) Human mtDNA and Y-chromosome variation is correlated with matrilocal versus patrilocal residence. *Nature Genetics*, **29**, 20–21.

72. Jobling, M.A. (2001) Y-chromosomal SNP haplotype diversity in forensic analysis. *Forensic Science International*, **118**, 158–162.

73. Jobling, M.A. (2001) In the name of the father: surnames and genetics. *Trends in Genetics*, **17**, 353–357.

74. Sykes, B. and Irven, C. (2000) Surnames and the Y chromosome. *American Journal of Human Genetics*, **66**, 1417–1419.

75. Gusmao, L., Butler, J.M., Carracedo, A., Gill, P., Kayser, M., Mayr, W.R. *et al.* (2006) DNA Commission of the International Society of Forensic Genetics (ISFG): an update of the recommendations on the use of Y-STRs in forensic analysis. *Forensic Sciences International*, **157**, 187–197.

76. Scientific Working Group on DNA Analysis Methods (2009) Y-chromosome short tandem repeat(Y STR) interpretation guidelines. *Forensic Science Communications*, **11** http://www.fbi.gov/hq/lab/fsc/backissu/jan2009/standards/2009_01_standards01.htm (accessed July 2010).

77. Kayser, M., Roewer, L., Hedman, M., Henke, L., Henke, J., Brauer, S. *et al.* (2000) Characteristics and frequency of germline mutations at microsatellite loci from the human Y chromosome, as revealed by direct observation in father/son pairs. *American Journal of Human Genetics*, **66**, 1580–1588.

78. Kayser, M. and Sajantila, A. (2001) Mutations at Y-STR loci: implications for paternity testing and forensic analysis. *Forensic Science International*, **118**, 116–121.

79. Gusmao, L., Sanchez-Diz, P., Calafell, F., Martin, P., Alonso, C.A., Alvarez-Fernandez, F. *et al.* (2005) Mutation rates at Y chromosome specific microsatellites. *Human Mutation*, **26**, 520–528.

80. Goedbloed, M., Vermeulen, M., Fang, R.N., Lembring, M., Wollstein, A., Ballantyne, K. *et al.* (2009) Comprehensive mutation analysis of 17 Y-chromosomal short tandem repeat polymorphisms included in the AmpFlSTR (R) Yfiler (R) PCR amplification kit. *International Journal of Legal Medicine*, **123**, 471–482.

81. Roewer, L. (2009) Y chromosome STR typing in crime casework. *Forensic Science, Medicine, and Pathology*, **5**, 77–84.

14 Non-human DNA typing

The use of DNA in human identification has dominated forensic science. The role of DNA has been to link a person to a person, a person to a scene and scenes to scenes. However, biological material from humans is only one component of the total DNA that can be encountered. Botanical and material from non-human animals are frequently recovered as part of the material examined in a forensic science laboratory, yet only rarely is this type of material analysed using genetic techniques. This chapter highlights the potential use of non-human DNA typing in forensic science.

Non-human sample types

Forensic cases where non-human DNA may be relevant fall into number of different categories.

Possession of protected species

There are an increasing number of species that are endangered and protected such that their possession is either contrary to international or national legislation. Examples of illegal materials include many hardwoods, curios made from protected tree species, animal skins, corals, ivory carvings and various products in traditional medicines (Figure 14.1). The Convention on the International Trade in Endangered Species of Flora and Fauna (CITES) is the international body that monitors the movement of endangered and protected species between countries that are members of CITES. The CITES enforcement team assist with international trade, but national legislation is required for wildlife crime within a country.

Crimes against people or property

Dogs and cats are common pets in many family homes and hairs from these pets are readily transferred on to the clothing of anyone entering such a home. A person entering into a car that is used to transport a dog may receive dog hairs on their clothing. Grass stains, leaf material and pollen grains are readily transferred from one location to another. Insect larvae feeding on a corpse can be difficult to identify, but DNA typing can identify the species present. The analysis of botanical material

An Introduction to Forensic Genetics Second Edition   William Goodwin, Adrian Linacre and Sibte Hadi
© 2011 John Wiley & Sons, Ltd

(a)   (b)

(c)

Figure 14.1 If illegal products are not highly processed, such as the tiger skins (a), then DNA evidence is not required for species identification, but make be required to match an individual skin with other evidence such as skeletal remains (b). (c) In other cases, such as the identification of threads from a shawl containing hairs from the Tibetan antelope (shatoosh) that is CITES listed, DNA analysis may be required to identify the fibres to a specific species (Images provided by Dr Surendra Goyal, Wildlife Institute of India, Chandrabani, India)

and other trace evidence such as hairs, feathers and larvae can provide a crucial link and act as associative evidence.

Crimes against animals

Cruelty to animals, illegal hunting, poaching and destruction of habitat are illegal activities in many countries that may lead to an investigation. DNA transferred from the animal to the human, the animal to an object or the human to the animal may provide the forensic evidence to support allegations of this type.

In the examples above there are two main questions that the forensic scientist should address: what species is this?, and do these two samples come from the same organism? Different types of tests are required to address these issues. The tests described in this chapter are all DNA-based. If there is morphology present then microscopy can, in certain circumstances, provide the answer to the questions above, but if the material is as a bloodstain or in trace amounts, then DNA typing offers the best opportunity to determine either a species or an individual organism.

Species identification

DNA typing has been used in taxonomy for the categorization of species. The same methods as used in this science can be utilized by forensic science. The locus of choice must have very little intraspecies variation, such that all members of the same species have the same DNA type. Equally, the locus used needs to have sufficient interspecies variation such that members of one species can be separated from members of the next closely related species. In animals, gene loci on the mitochondrial genome fit these criteria best, primarily as mitochondria do not contain an error reading enzyme to repair DNA bases added incorrectly during DNA replication [1]. As such, mitochondrial DNA mutates five times faster than nuclear DNA. The analysis of genes on the mitochondria also has the advantages of being present at very high copy number [2].

The mitochondrial locus used most commonly in taxonomy and forensic science is the cytochrome *b* gene. The human cytochrome *b* gene lies at position 14 756–15 896, adjacent to the hypervariable region I (HVI) (see Figure 13.1). In all mammalian species, this gene lies in the same position but because of the variation in the size of mammalian species its base position alters. It encodes a protein, 380 amino acids in length, involved in the oxidative process of respiration. DNA sequences for over 8000 different species have been decoded and registered with one of the DNA databases, such as EMBL (www.ebi.ac.uk) or GenBank (www.ncbi.nlm.nih.gov). The complete gene is 1140 bases in length and too large for standard PCR-based amplification, especially from forensic evidence that is often degraded. As this is a gene for an enzyme used in respiration, parts of the protein are under selection pressure, and therefore similar in a large number of diverse species. An example of a sequence alignment is shown in Figure 14.2. This allows the development of primer sets that will work on all mammalian species. The DNA sequences between the conserved regions shows sufficient variation such that members of closely related

```
Consensus     GCTCCCTACTAGGAATCTGCCTAATCTTACAAATCCTAACCGGACTATTC
Indian Rhino.......GT..........T.........G........A..........
Javan Rhino .........T...........T.........G.....G..A..........
White Rhino .......G...........T............T..............
Black Rhino ....T....................C....................T
Sumatran      ..................................................
Unknown 1     .......G...........T...........T................
Unknown 2     .......G...........T...........T................
Unknown 3     ....T....................C....................T
Unknown 4     ....T....................C....................T
Unknown 5     ....T....................C....................T
```

Figure 14.2 Showing an alignment of 50 bp within the cyt *b* gene for the four extant species of rhino (Black and White live in Africa and the Indian, Java and Sumatra are the Asian relatives) compared to five bone samples of unknown species. Unknown 1 and 2 have a 100% match to the White Rhino and Unknown 3, 4 and 5 are the same and are a 100% match to the Black Rhino species can be distinguished but members of the same species have the same (or nearly the same) DNA sequence.

The process of species identification is relatively straightforward [3]. DNA is isolated from the unknown material and amplification primers are used to produce a PCR product of around 400 bp in length [4, 5]. This product is sequenced and the DNA sequence is compared with those on the DNA database. If there is a 100% match to a DNA sequence from a registered species, and the next closest species has a homology of 95%, then there is every reason to believe that the unknown material is from the species to which it matched.

Another mitochondrial locus used in species testing in the cytochrome oxidase 1 gene. This locus is promoted by the Barcode for Life consortium [6] and is used in exactly the same way as cytochrome *b*, only a section of 648 bp is used for the comparison. Both the cytochrome *b* gene and the cytochrome oxidase 1 gene have been used successfully in species identification.

There are numerous examples of species identification in forensic science: these include the identification of tiger DNA within traditional medicines [7]; protected bear species in bear bile products [8]; rhino DNA smuggled as bovine bone [9]; turtles as food products and as shell ornaments [10]; identification of elephant ivory within statues [11]; protected shark species collected for shark fin soup [12, 13]; the identification of the Tibetan antelope on woven shawls [14]; and the identification of cannabis from seeds [15].

In green plants, loci on the chloroplast DNA are used more commonly for species identification. The loci include *matK* and *trnH -psbA* [16], the transfer RNA (tRNA) genes [17], the internal transcribed spacer (ITS) regions in ribosomal RNA (rRNA) [18, 19] and genes such as ribulose 1,5 bis-phosphate carboxylase (*rbcL*), ATP synthase beta (*atpB*) and the NADH dehydrogenase subunit 5 (*ndhF*) [20]. In the case of the *rbcL* locus over 6500 plant species have so far been examined. Although this is a large number, it represents a fraction of the actual plant species known. The complexity of genomes within the plant kingdom reflects the large number of loci used in species identification.

Linkage to an individual using STR loci

Plants and animals contain STRs, similar to those described in Chapter 6. The human STR loci were identified and characterized as they are often intron based and were discovered while examining the gene sequences. Although all animal and plant species contain STRs, they have only been characterized to any great extent in commercially important species such as dog [21–23], cat [24–26], horse [27, 28], cow [29], pigeons [30], pine trees [31, 32] and cannabis [33–36]. STR loci are only useful if there is a database of alleles for comparison. There are databases in place for the species listed above. Originally the STR loci identified were predominantly dinucleotide repeats, but with the increasing knowledge of the genomes of domesticated species, tetranucleotide repeats are more common.

The first case that highlighted the use of animal STR typing was that of Snowball the cat. In this case a bloodstained jacket was found next to the body of a female. White hairs were noted on the jacket and identified as being from a cat. The estranged husband of the deceased denied any knowledge of the jacket, but a white cat called Snowball shared the home where the husband stayed. Ten feline STRs were tested on a sample from Snowball and the hair from the jacket and found to match. Population studies on nearby cats indicated a high power of discrimination using these 10 STR loci and led to the conviction of the husband [37]. Since then there have been cases of dog STR typing, to link dog hairs to a living dog [38]. These types of analyses are used to link a non-human DNA to an investigation of an alleged crime against a person.

Crimes against animals include badger baiting, where dogs are set on wild badgers. STR loci have been developed to link badger blood and hairs from items retrieved from anyone alleged to have been present at such an act to a deceased badger [39]. Other uses of STR typing are to link offspring of birds of prey to the hen and cock bird, as it is permissible to own a bird if bred from captive pairs rather than taken from the wild [40, 41]. If a person claims that a bird of prey in their possession was bred from captive stock, then this can be tested.

Botanical uses of STR typing include the linkage of leaf material within a car to an oak tree growing at the site of a shallow grave [42]. In this case four oak STR loci were found to match between the leaf and reference material from the tree, with a match probability of 2.06×10^{-6}. Many more such botanical cases could be performed if there were more comprehensive reference databases available.

Adjustment of allele frequencies from human DNA databases was discussed in Chapter 8. The same process should be undertaken with non-human STR data. Rare or absent alleles need to be accounted for either by the application of a minimal allele frequency, or the addition of the unknown and known alleles to the database followed by a recalculation. Kinship factors can be a problem with breeds, or where there are very small populations remaining and species that reproduce colonially. In these cases a knowledge of the biology of the species is needed such that an appropriate kinship factor is applied to the alleles when determining the overall genotype frequency.

Linkage to an individual using mitochondrial loci

Non-human material is often a fine animal hair, in which case there is insufficient genetic material to obtain an STR profile. Examination of the control region of the mitochondrial DNA can be conducted in much the same way as the sequence comparison of HVI and HVII as described for human linkage. Mitochondrial control databases exist for dog [43–45] to allow an estimate of the chance that another dog might have the same DNA type. The power of discrimination will be less using mitochondrial sequence data than using STR analysis; however, these data can still be of value as associative evidence.

Microbial DNA testing

The DNA typing of microbes in forensic science can be either for bioterrorism [46, 47] or for the comparison of soils [48]. Undoubtedly the possibility of being able to link soil samples based on their DNA profile would allow even more biological material to be examined than at present. The problem at present is that it is difficult to reproduce the same result from soil samples.

Concluding comments

Two main questions are asked with non-human DNA: what species is this and from which particular organism did it originate? Species testing using either mitochondrial gene loci or those on the chloroplast has become routine, but is dependent on the species in question being registered on one of the sequence databases. The success of STR typing of non-human DNA samples is dependent on the primer sites either side of the STR being known, and the appropriate evaluation of the data is dependent on knowledge of the biology of the species when considering the chance that the DNA comes from any other member of the same species.

As the use of DNA typing from human samples has become routine, it is not surprising that there is an ever-increasing interest in using similar methods on non-human samples. The examinations are performed either by forensic science laboratories with little knowledge of species other than humans, or by universities with a knowledge of the biology of the species but little knowledge of forensic science. The optimum is where the testing is performed by those with both knowledge of the species concerned and a forensic science background.

Further reading

Coyle, H. (ed.) (2008) *Nonhuman DNA Typing*, International Forensic Science and Investigation Series, CRC Press, Boca Raton.
Linacre, A. (ed.) (2009) *Forensic Science in Wildlife Investigations*, International Forensic Science and Investigation Series, CRC Press, Boca Raton.

WWW resources

CITES Secretariat: http://www.cites.org/
United Nations Environment Programme: World Conservation Monitoring Centre http://www.unep-wcmc.org/
Interpol: http://www.interpol.int/Public/EnvironmentalCrime/Wildlife/Default.asp

References

1. Gray, M.W. (1989) Origin and evolution of mitochondrial-DNA. *Annual Review of Cell Biology*, **5**, 25–50.
2. Satoh, M. and Kuroiwa, T. (1991) Organization of multiple nucleoids and DNA-molecules in mitochondria of a human cell. *Experimental Cell Research*, **196**, 137–140.

3. Linacre, A. and Lee, J.C.-I. (2005) Species identification: the role of the cytochrome b gene, in *Forensic DNA Typing Protocols* (ed. A. Carracedo), Humana Press, pp. 45–53.

4. Hsieh, H.-M., Chiang, H.-L., Tsai, L.-C., Lai, S.-Y., Huang, N.-E. and Linacre, A. *et al.* (2001) Cytochrome b gene for species identification of the conservation animals. *Forensic Science International*, **122**, 7–18.

5. Irwin, D., Kocher, T. and Wilson, A. (1991) Evolution of the cytochrome b gene of mammals. *Journal of Molecular Evolution*, **32**, 128–144.

6. Hebert, P.D.N. Ratnasingham S, de Waard JR. (2003) Barcoding animal life: cytochrome c oxidase subunit 1 divergences among closely related species. *Proceedings of the Royal Society of London. Series B: Biological Sciences*, **270**, S96–S99.

7. Wetton, J.H., Tsang, C.S.F., Roney, C.A.and Spriggs, A.C. (2004) An extremely sensitive species-specific ARMs PCR test for the presence of tiger bone DNA. *Forensic Science International*, **140**, 139–145.

8. Peppin, L., McEwing, R., Carvalho, G.R. and Ogden, R. (2008) A DNA-based approach for the forensic identification of Asiatic black bear (Ursus thibetanus) in a traditional Asian medicine. *Journal of Forensic Sciences*, **53**, 1358–1362.

9. Hsieh, H.-M., Huang, L.-H., Tsai, L.-C., Kuo, Y.-C., Meng, H.-H., Linacre, A. *et al.* (2003) Species identification of rhinoceros horns using the cytochrome b gene. *Forensic Science International*, **136**, 1–11.

10. Lee, J.C.I., Tsai, L.C., Liao, S.P., Linacre, A. and Hsieh, H.M. (2009) Species identification using the cytochrome b gene of commercial turtle shells. *Forensic Science International Genetics*, **3**, 67–73.

11. Lee, J., Hsieh, H.M., Huang, L.H., Kuo, Y.C., Wu, J.H. and Chin, S.C. (2009) Ivory identification by DNA profiling of cytochrome b gene. *International Journal of Legal Medicine*, **123**, 117–121.

12. Chapman, D.D., Abercrombie, D.L., Douady, C.J., Pikitch, E.K., Stanhopen, M.J. and Shivji, M.S. (2003) A streamlined, bi-organelle, multiplex PCR approach to species identification: application to global conservation and trade monitoring of the great white shark, Carcharodon carcharias. *Conservation Genetics*, **4**, 415–425.

13. Shivji, M., Clarke, S., Pank, M., Natanson, L., Kohler, N. and Stanhope, M. (2002) Genetic identification of pelagic shark body parts for conservation and trade monitoring. *Conservation Biology*, **16**, 1036–1047.

14. Lee, J.C.I., Tsai, L.C., Yang, C.Y., Liu, C.L., Huang, L.H. and Linacre, A. (2006) DNA profiling of shahtoosh. *Electrophoresis*, **27**, 3359–3362.

15. Tsai, L.C., Hsieh, H.M., Wang, J.C., Huang, L.H., Linacre, A. and Lee, J.C.I. (2006) Cannabis seed identification by chloroplast and nuclear DNA. *Forensic Science International*, **158**, 250–251.

16. Kress, W.J., Wurdack, K.J., Zimmer, E.A., Weigt, L.A. and Janzen, D.H. (2005) Use of DNA barcodes to identify flowering plants. *Proceedings of the National Academy of Sciences of the United States of America.*, **102**, 8369–8374.

17. Tsai, L.C., Yu, Y.C., Hsieh, H.M., Wang, J.C., Linacre, A. and Lee, J.C.I. (2006) Species identification using sequences of the trnL intron and the trnL-trnF IGS of chloroplast genome among popular plants in Taiwan. *Forensic Science International*, **164**, 193–200.

18. Tsai, L.C., Wang, J.C., Hsieh, H.M., Liu, K.L., Linacre, A. and Lee, J.C.I. (2008) Bidens identification using the noncoding regions of chloroplast genome and nuclear ribosomal DNA. *Forensic Science International Genetics*, **2**, 35–40.

19. Gigliano, G.S. (1999) Preliminary data on the usefulness of Internal Transcribed Spacer I (ITS1) sequence in Cannabis sativa L. identification. *Journal of Forensic Sciences*, **44**, 475–477.

20. Soltis, D.E., Soltis, P.S. and Doyle, J.J. (eds) (1998) *Systematics of Plants II*, Kluwer Academic Publishers.

21. Dayton, M., Koskinen, M.T., Tom, B.K., Mattila, A.M., Johnston, E. and Halverson, J. (2009) Developmental validation of short tandem repeat reagent kit for forensic DNA profiling of canine biological material. *Croatian Medical Journal*, **50**, 268–285.

22. Kanthaswamy, S., Tom, B.K., Mattila, A.M., Johnston, E., Dayton, M. and Kinaga, J. (2009) Canine population data generated from a multiplex STR kit for use in forensic casework. *Journal of Forensic Sciences*, **54**, 829–840.

23. van Asch, B., Alves, C., Gusmao, L., Pereira, V., Pereira, F. and Amorim A. (2009) A new autosomal STR nineplex for canine identification and parentage testing. *Electrophoresis*, **30**, 417–423.

24. Berger, B., Eichmann, C. and Parson, W. (2008) Forensic canine STR analysis, in *Nonhuman DNA Typing* (ed. H. Coyle), CRC Press, pp. 45–68.

25. Coomber, N., David, V.A., O'Brien, S.J. and Menotti-Raymond, M. (2007) Validation of a short tandem repeat multiplex typing system for genetic individualization of domestic cat samples. *Croatian Medical Journal*, **48**, 547–555.

26. Menotti-Raymond, M.A., David, V.A., Wachter, L.L., Butler, J.M. and O'Brien, S.J. (2005) An STIR forensic typing system for genetic individualization of domestic cat (Felis catus) samples. *Journal of Forensic Sciences*, **50**, 1061–1070.

27. Bowling, A.T., EgglestonStott, M.L., Byrns, G., Clark, R.S., Dileanis, S. and Wictum, E. (1997) Validation of microsatellite markers for routine horse parentage testing. *Animal Genetics*, **28**, 247–252.

28. Dimsoski, P. (2003) Development of a 17-plex microsatellite polymerase chain reaction kit for genotyping horses. *Croatian Medical Journal*, **44**, 332–335.

29. van de Goor, L.H.P., Panneman, H. and van Haeringen, W.A. (2009) A proposal for standardization in forensic bovine DNA typing: allele nomenclature of 16 cattle-specific short tandem repeat loci. *Animal Genetics*, **40**, 630–636.

30. Chun-Lee, J., Tsai, L.C., Kuan, Y.Y., Chien, W.H., Chang, K.T., Wu, C.H. *et al.* (2007) Racing pigeon identification using STR and chromo-helicase DNA binding gene markers. *Electrophoresis*, **28**, 4274–4281.

31. Marquardt, P.E. and Epperson, B.K. (2004) Spatial and population genetic structure of microsatellites in white pine. *Molecular Ecology*, **13**, 3305–3315.

32. Slavov, G.T., Howe, G.T., Yakovlev, I., Edwards, K.J., Krutovskii, K.V., Tuskan, G.A. *et al.* (2004) Highly variable SSR markers in Douglas-fir: Mendelian inheritance and map locations. *Theoretical and Applied Genetics*, **108**, 873–880.

33. Howard, C., Gilmore, S., Robertson, J. and Peakall, R. (2008) Developmental validation of a Cannabis sativa STIR multiplex system for forensic analysis. *Journal of Forensic Sciences*, **53**, 1061–1067.

34. Howard, C., Gilmore, S., Robertson, J. and Peakall, R. (2009) A Cannabis sativa STR genotype database for Australian seizures: forensic applications and limitations. *Journal of Forensic Sciences*, **54**, 556–563.

35. Hsieh, H.M., Hou, R.J., Tsai, L.C., Wei, C.S., Liu, S.W., Huang, L.H. *et al.* (2003) A highly polymorphic STR locus in Cannabis sativa. *Forensic Science International*, **131**, 53–58.

36. Mendoza, M.A., Mills, D.K., Lata, H., Chandra, S., ElSohly, M.A. and Almirall, J.R. (2009) Genetic individualization of Cannabis sativa by a short tandem repeat multiplex system. *Analytical and Bioanalytical Chemistry*, **393**, 719–726.

37. Menotti-Raymond, M., David, V. and O'Brien, S. (1997) Pet cat hair implicates murder suspect. *Nature*, **386**, 774.

38. Halverson, J.L. and Basten, C. (2005) Forensic DNA identification of animal-derived trace evidence: tools for linking victims and suspects. *Croatian Medical Journal*, **46**, 598–605.

39. Dawnay, N., Ogden, R., Thorpe, R.S., Pope, L.C., Dawson, D.A. and McEwing, R. (2008) A forensic STR profiling system for the Eurasian badger: a framework for developing profiling systems for wildlife species. *Forensic Science International Genetics*, **2**, 47–53.

40. Dawnay, N., McEwing, R., Thorpe, R.S. and Ogden, R. (2008) Preliminary data suggests genetic distinctiveness of gyr and saker falcons. *Conservation Genetics*, **9**, 703–707.

41. Dawnay, N., Ogden, R., Wetton, J.H., Thorpe, R.S. and McEwing, R. (2009) Genetic data from 28 STR loci for forensic individual identification and parentage analyses in 6 bird of prey species. *Forensic Science International Genetics*, **3**, e63–e69.

42. Craft, K.J., Owens, J.D. and Ashley, M.V. (2007) Application of plant DNA markers in forensic botany: genetic comparison of Quercus evidence leaves to crime scene trees using microsatellites. *Forensic Science International*, **165**, 64–70.

43. Gundry, R.L., Allard, M.W., Moretti, T.R., Honeycutt, R.L., Wilson, M.R. and Monson, K.L. (2007) Mitochondrial DNA analysis of the domestic dog: control region variation within and among breeds. *Journal of Forensic Sciences*, **52**, 562–572.

44. Himmelberger, A.L., Spear, T.F., Satkoski, J.A., George, D.A., Garnica, W.T. and Malladi, V.S. (2008) Forensic utility of the mitochondrial hypervariable region 1 of domestic dogs, in conjunction with breed and geographic information. *Journal of Forensic Sciences*, **53**, 81–89.

45. Webb, K.M. and Allard, M.W. (2009) Identification of forensically informative SNPs in the domestic dog mitochondrial control region. *Journal of Forensic Sciences*, **54**, 289–304.

46. Budowle, B., Beaudry, J.A., Barnaby, N.G., Giusti, A.M., Bannan, J.D. and Keim, P. (2007) Role of law enforcement response and microbial forensics in investigation of bioterrorism. *Croatian Medical Journal*, **48**, 437–449.

47. Morse, S.A. and Budowle, B. (2006) Microbial forensics: application to bioterrorism preparedness and response. *Infectious Disease Clinics of North America*, **20**, 455–445.

48. Heath, L.E. and Saunders, V.A. (2006) Assessing the potential of bacterial DNA profiling for forensic soil comparisons. *Journal of Forensic Sciences*, **51**, 1062–1068.

Appendix A Forensic parameters

Match probability

The probability that the two randomly selected individuals within a population will have identical genotypes at a locus.

Formula:

$$p_M = \sum_{k=1}^{m} p_k^2$$

where p_M is the match probability of individual locus, p_k represents the frequency of each distinct genotype that is possible (which in turn depends on the number of alleles at the locus), m is the number of the distinctive genotypes.

Power of discrimination

The probability that two randomly selected individuals will have different genotypes.

Formulae:

For a single locus the formula is: $p_D = 1 - p_M$

For several loci the formula is: $P_{Dcomb} = 1 - \prod_{i=1}^{n}(1 - P_{Di})$

where, p_D is the power of discrimination of a single locus, p_M is the match probability of a single locus, P_{Dcomb} is the power of discrimination of several loci, P_{Di} is the individual locus power of discrimination and $\prod$ stands for multiplication.

Power of exclusion

Is the fraction of the individuals that is different from that of a randomly selected individual. It can also be defined as the power of a locus to exclude a person being

An Introduction to Forensic Genetics Second Edition William Goodwin, Adrian Linacre and Sibte Hadi
© 2011 John Wiley & Sons, Ltd

the biological father. Thus the value differs in each case. The average for a locus is the power for a single locus.

Formulae:

$$PE = h^2(1 - 2hH^2)$$

where h is the heterozygosity and H is the homozygosity at the locus.

For several loci the formula is:

$$PE_{comb} = 1 - \prod_{l=1}^{L}(1 - PE_l)$$

where L is the number of the loci, PE_l is the exclusion probability for the l_{th} locus and Π stands for multiplication.

Polymorphic information content

Indicates the polymorphic level of a locus.

Formula:

$$PIC = 1 - \sum_{i=1}^{n}pi^2 - \left(\sum_{i=1}^{n}pi^2\right)^2 + \sum_{i=1}^{n}pi^4$$

where pi is the frequency of each distinct allele and n is the number of distinct alleles.

Appendix B Useful web links

Professional bodies and agencies

ANZFSS – The Australian and New Zealand Forensic Science Society, Inc. http://www.anzfss.org.au/index.htm.

ENSFI – European Network of Forensic Science Institutes. http://www.enfsi.org/.

FBI – Federal Bureau of Investigation: FBI Laboratory. http://www.fbi.gov/hq/lab/labhome.htm.

FSS – The Forensic Science Service (UK). http://www.forensic.gov.uk/.

ISFG – International Society for Forensic Genetics: http://www.isfg.org/.

INTERPOL – The International Criminal Police Organization. http://www.interpol.int/.

NIFS – National Institute of Forensic Science Australia. http://www.nifs.com.au/home.html.

The Forensic Science Society (UK). http://www.forensic-science-society.org.uk/.

Statistical analysis

Forensic Mathematics: Contains information of the kinship software with DNA·View™ and articles/discussions focused on the statistical/mathematical interpretation of DNA profiles. http://dna-view.com.

GDA: a statistical software package that computes linkage and Hardy–Weinberg disequilibrium, some genetic distances and provides method-of-moments estimators for hierarchical F-statistics. http://hydrodictyon.eeb.uconn.edu/people/plewis/software.php.

Powerstats: A Microsoft Office Excel-based tool for calculating descriptive statistics and forensic parameters for STR loci. http://www.promega.com/geneticidtools/powerstats/.

An Introduction to Forensic Genetics Second Edition   William Goodwin, Adrian Linacre and Sibte Hadi
© 2011 John Wiley & Sons, Ltd

ENFSI DNA WG STR Population Database: calculates the profile frequency of a SGM Plus profile using 24 European allele frequency databases. http://www.str-base.org/index.php.

Genetic markers and population databases

STRBase – Short Tandem Repeat DNA Internet DataBase: contains a large amount of information on STR polymorphisms. http://www.cstl.nist.gov/biotech/strbase/.

YHRD – Y Chromosome Haplotype Reference Database: a searchable database of Y chromosome STR haplotypes. http://www.yhrd.org.

EMPOP – Mitochondrial DNA Control Region Database: a collection of searchable mtDNA control region haplotypes from all over the world. http://www.empop.org/.

MITOMAP – A compendium of polymorphisms and mutations of the human mitochondrial DNA. http://www.mitomap.org/.

ALFRED – The ALlele FREquency Database: contains allele frequency data for a wide range of genetic polymorphisms in different populations. http://alfred.med.yale.edu/.

Commercial providers

All these companies provide a wide range of products in addition to the ones noted.

Applied Biosystems: suppliers of kits and equipment for the analysis of STR and SNP polymorphisms. http://www.appliedbiosystems.com/.

Promega Corporation: suppliers of kits for STR analysis and a wide variety of molecular biology products. http://www.promega.com/.

Qiagen: suppliers of widely used DNA isolation kits. http://www1.qiagen.com/.

Whatman®: suppliers of FTA® card. http://www.whatman.com/.

Glossary

Allele: alternative forms of a gene or section of DNA at a given genetic locus.

Allelic Drop Out: non-detection of an allele at a given locus. This results in only one of the two alleles being detected at a heterozygous locus.

Allelic Ladder: a mixture of all the common alleles at a given locus. The allelic ladder allows comparison with the unknown alleles and assists in allelic designation.

Amplifiable Fragment Length Polymorphisms (AMP-FLPs): polymorphic loci where alleles differ in the number of tandem core repeats. Alleles are typically between 500 bp and 1000 bp in length. An example of an AMP-FLP is the locus D1S80.

Autosome: a non-sex chromosome. In humans there are the 22 pairs of autosomal chromosomes; these do not include the X and Y sex chromosomes.

bp: base pair – two complementary nucleotides in double-stranded DNA. Adenine pairs with thymine and guanine pairs with cytosine.

Chromosome: a single molecule of double-stranded DNA associated with proteins to form a highly ordered structure. Chromosomes are located in the cell nucleus of eukaryotes and are visible with light microscopy only during cell division when they become highly condensed.

CODIS loci: the FBI defined a set of 13 STR markers for use in forensic analysis.

Diploid: presence of two sets of chromosomes in a cell and therefore containing two copies of the genome.

DNA polymerase: an enzyme that catalyses the formation of a complementary DNA strand in the $5'-3'$ direction acting on a template DNA strand.

Electrophoresis: separation of charged molecules through a matrix. DNA is negatively charged and will migrate from the cathode (−ve) to the anode (+ve) when an electric current is applied across the matrix.

Euchromatin: part of the chromosome that is loosely packed in the interphase of the cell cycle. Most of the transcribed regions of the genome are located within the euchromatin.

Gene: a functional part of DNA that encodes a protein or RNA molecule.

Gene Frequency: the relative frequency (proportion) of a gene in a population.

Genome: the entire haploid complement of DNA in a cell or organism. The human genome comprises approximately 3.2 billion bp.

Genotype: the particular set of alleles present in each cell. At any one locus the two alleles define the genotype such that if there are only two alleles then there are three possible genotypes (AA, AB, BB).

Haploid: presence of one set of chromosomes in a cell and therefore containing one copy of the genome. Cells such as egg cells and spermatozoa carry a haploid genome and the Y chromosome and mitochondrial DNA are haploid.

Hardy–Weinberg Law (HW law): a law stating that in an ideal population, the frequencies of an allele will remain constant from one generation to the next.

Heterochromatin: a highly condensed part of the chromosome which remains tightly packed throughout the cell cycle and is predominantly non-coding.

Heterozygous: having different alleles at any particular locus.

Homozygous: presence of two identical alleles at a given locus.

Locus: the physical position of a gene or section of DNA on a chromosome. The plural of locus is loci.

Locus Drop Out: the non-detection of both alleles at a given locus.

Low Copy Number PCR: a more sensitive method of DNA profiling where the number of cycles is increased in order to amplify amounts of DNA typically less than 100 pg.

Low Template DNA PCR: any process that aims to increase the sensitivity of DNA testing in order to amplify amounts of DNA typically less than 100 pg.

Mitochondria: small semi-autonomous organelles of the cell which are primarily responsible for energy production. They have their own circular genome that is 16 569 bp in length in humans.

Mutation: alteration in the DNA sequence. The most common form of a mutation is a single base transition (see next page).

Oligonucleotide: a short sequence of single-stranded DNA.

Phenotype: physical form of an organism resulting from genetic traits and environmental factors.

Polymerase Chain Reaction (PCR): a process of enzymatic amplification of DNA *in vitro*.

Posterior Odds: in terms of a court case these are the odds of guilt of a defendant after the presentation of all evidence. It is the posterior odds that the judge or jury consider when coming to a verdict.

Primer: oligonuclceotide that binds to complementary single-stranded DNA and acts as a priming site for the initiation for the synthesis of the complementary strand by DNA polymerase.

Prior Odds: in terms of a court case these are the odds of guilt of a defendant before the presentation of forensic evidence and may be considered as based on the non-scientific evidence.

Purine: nitrogenous bases found in nucleic acids. The purine bases are adenine and guanine.

Pyrimidine: nitrogenous bases found in nucleic acids. The pyrimidine bases are cytosine and thymine.

Restriction Enzyme: enzyme with endonucleic activity that cuts DNA at specific sequences. An example is *Eco*RI that cuts within the sequence GAATTC.

Restriction Fragment Length Polymorphism: the detection of length or sequence variation after cleaving DNA with a restriction enzyme (see above), separating on a gel, transferring to a membrane by Southern blotting (see below) and detection using a small section of DNA within the sequence between two restriction sites. RFLP testing was used in the detection of minisatellites.

Short Tandem Repeat (STR): polymorphic region of DNA where alleles differ in the number of tandemly arranged core repeats. STR alleles typically range in size between 100 bp and 400 bp. Also known as microsatellites.

Single Nucleotide Polymorphism (SNP): the occurrence of two (or more) alleles at a single base position within the genome. SNPs are typically biallelic: transitions (see below) are more common than transversions (see next page). To be considered as a population level SNP polymorphism the rare allele should be at a frequency greater than 1%.

Southern Blot: a technique that is used to transfer DNA from a gel onto a nylon membrane.

Telomere: the terminal regions at the tips of the chromosomes. Satellite DNA forms much of the telomeric regions.

Theta (θ) Statistic: a measurement of inbreeding within a population. Theta is often used interchangeably with F_{ST} in forensic genetics.

Transition: the change in a base from a purine (see above) to a purine (A/G) or a pyrimidine to a pyrimidine (C/T).

Transversion: the change in a base from a purine to a pyrimidine (A or G to C or T) or a pyrimidine to a purine (C or T to A or G).

Variable Number Tandem Repeat (VNTR): polymorphic region of DNA where alleles differ in the number of tandemly arranged core repeats. VNTR alleles can range in size from around 500 bp to over 20 kb. Also known as minisatellites.

Abbreviations

ALAS2: δ-aminolevulinate synthase

ALS: Alternative light source

AMP-FLP: amplified fragment length polymorphism

ASO: allele-specific oligonucleotide

atpB: ATP synthase beta

BSA: bovine serum albumin

CCD: charged coupled device

CE: capillary electrophoresis

CGE: capillary gel electrophoresis

CITES: Convention on the International Trade in Endangered Species
of Flora and Fauna

CODIS: Combined DNA Index System

CRS: Cambridge Reference Sequence

DAPI: 4′,6-diamidino-2-phenylindole

ddNTP: dideoxyribonucleotide triphosphate

dNTP: deoxynucleotide triphosphate

DTT: dithiothreitol

ECHR: European Court of Human Rights

EDTA: ethylene-diamine tetraacetic acid

ENFSI: European Network of Forensic Science Institutes

ESS: European Standard Set

FSS: Forensic Science Service (UK)

HLA: human leukocyte antigen

An Introduction to Forensic Genetics Second Edition   William Goodwin, Adrian Linacre and Sibte Hadi

HV: hypervariable

HWE: Hardy–Weinberg equilibrium

HW: Hardy–Weinberg

ISSOL: Interpol Standard Set of Loci

ITS: internal transcribed spacer

KM: Kastle–Mayer

LCN: low copy number

LDIS: Local DNA Index System

LINE: long interspersed element

LMG: leucomalachite green

LR: likelihood ratio

LTR: long terminal repeat

MGB: minor groove binder

MHC: major histocompatibility complex

MLP: multi-locus probe

MMP-7: matrix metalloproteinase-7

mRNA: messenger RNA

NCBI dbSNP: National Center for Biotechnology Information SNP database

ndhF: NADH dehydrogenase subunit 5

NDIS: National DNA Index System

NDNAD: National DNA Database

OL: off-ladder

PACE: Police and Criminal Evidence

PAR: pseudoautosomal region

PBGD: porphobilinogen deaminase

PCR: polymerase chain reaction

PI: paternity index

PRM: protamine

PSA: prostate-specific antigen

rbcL: ribulose 1,5 bis-phosphate carboxylase

RFU: relative fluorescent units

rRNA: ribosomal RNA

SAP: seminal acid phosphatase

SBE: single-base extension

SDIS: State DNA Index System

SDS: sodium dodecyl sulphate

SGM: second generation multiplex

SINE: short interspersed element

SLP: single locus probe

SNP: single nucleotide polymorphism

SPTB: β-spectrin

SRY: sex determining region Y

STR: short tandem repeat

TC: tested child

TMB: tetramethylbenzidine

tRNA: transfer RNA

UD: undisputed

VNTR: variable number tandem repeat

yhrd: Y Chromosome Haplotype Reference Database

Units of measurement

Prefix	Symbol	10^n	Numerical representation
giga	G	10^9	1 000 000 000
mega	M	10^6	1 000 000
kilo	k	10^3	1 000
milli	m	10^{-3}	0.001
micro	μ	10^{-6}	0.000 001
nano	n	10^{-9}	0.000 000 001
pico	p	10^{-12}	0.000 000 000 001

Index